"One of the keys to happiness is remembering to laugh, and Dr. Dana reminds us frequently of how to do that in *The Top Ten Lies We Tell Ourselves*. She's not just joking around, though, because she knows her stuff. She connects the most important principles of A *Course in Miracles* to her knowledge of psychology and then makes it clear that she's really used both in her own life. After this book, lying to myself won't be such a big deal anymore!"

—Maria Felipe, author of *Live Your Happy*

"Dr. Dana Marrocco's beautifully written guide through the ego's biggest lies is a heavenly compass for spiritual progress. Grounded in psychology and academic research, *The Top Ten Lies We Tell Ourselves* invites the reader to walk through an internal process of compassionate self-awareness to turn our fearful perceptions on their heads and return to a high-voltage perception of love. Dr. Dana's series of exercises take us beyond the limitations of our conditioning and fear-based mental hooks to a brighter experience of life."

—Lyna Rose, author of *Enlighten Your Life*

"*The Top Ten Lies We Tell Ourselves* is a humorous look at the upside-down, fearful thought system of the ego part of our mind. By exposing our most common but not-so-obvious beliefs, this book will help you shift your mind to a right-side-up way of thinking, thereby freeing your mind from fear and setting you on a path of peace. The exercises throughout facilitate this awakening, and the twenty-four-hour challenges are brilliant!"

—Corinne Zupko, EdS, author of *From Anxiety to Love*

"Open this book, begin to read, and see if you can't find the truth, which will make you free. According to A *Course in Miracles*, we do not perceive our own best interests and need clarity to better understand what those interests are. This is an overall theme in Dr. Dana's conscientiously written book, reinforcing the practice of looking inward with total honesty to experience the happiness we deserve."

—Jon Mundy, PhD, author of *Living* A *Course in Miracles*

"Dr. Dana's voice speaks to me exactly where it helps most. She points to the hidden traps I have fallen into and how I can reverse my addictive beliefs that led me down the rabbit hole. The reader can easily identify with the 'ten lies' we grew up with, mistakes that weaken us and will persist until we change our mind. I recommend this book to anyone who chooses to see things differently and stop living the mistakes of the past."

—H. David Fishman, author of *Into Oneness*

THE TOP TEN
LIES
WE TELL
OURSELVES

For Barbara,

Be the love...

Dr. Dana

THE TOP TEN LIES WE TELL OURSELVES

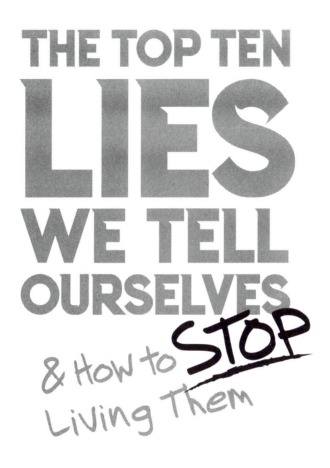

& How to STOP Living Them

DR. DANA MARROCCO

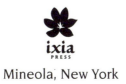

ixia PRESS

Mineola, New York

Bibliographical Note

The Top Ten Lies We Tell Ourselves—And How to Stop Living Them is a new work, first published by Ixia Press in 2018.

Acknowledgments

All quotes from A *Course in Miracles* are from the Third Edition, published in 2007. They are used with written permission from the copyright holder and publisher, the Foundation for Inner Peace, PO Box 598, Mill Valley, California 94942-0598, www.acim.org and info@acim.org.

Library of Congress Cataloging-in-Publication Data

Names: Marrocco, Dana, author.
Title: The top ten lies we tell ourselves : and how to stop living them / Dr. Dana Marrocco.
Description: Mineola, New York : Ixia Press, 2018. I Includes bibliographical references and index.
Identifiers: LCCN 2018007301I ISBN 9780486821542 (alk. paper) I ISBN 0486821544 (alk. paper)
Subjects: LCSH: Self-deception. I Self-perception
Classification: LCC BF697.5.S426 M37 2018 I DDC 158.1—dc23
LC record available at https://lccn.loc.gov/2018007301

Ixia Press
An imprint of Dover Publications, Inc.

Manufactured in the United States by LSC Communications
82154401   2018
www.doverpublications.com/ixiapress

I dedicate this book to my husband and children—
the greatest symbols of love I could have imagined.

CONTENTS

FOREWORD

I first met Dr. Dana several years ago when I went to the Unity Spiritual Center in Pattenburg, New Jersey, to give a Sunday afternoon workshop. I also was scheduled to speak at the Sunday morning church service, and an old friend of mine, John Beavin, was there to supply the music along with several other members of the regular church band. Dana was part of it, and they had humorously given the group the name Dr. Dana and the Infinite Patients. I liked that name a lot. If there's one thing we need more of in the realm of spirituality, it's humor.

When I found out that Dana was a psychologist, I was a bit standoffish, because I thought she'd probably figure out pretty quickly everything that was wrong with me. Still, I enjoyed the music and the day very much. A few of us, including Dana, went out for dinner after, where she and I started to get to know each other better.

As the years went by, Dana and I would exchange e-mails about our chosen spiritual path, A *Course in Miracles* (also called ACIM or simply the *Course*), and I'd see enlightening videos that she did on YouTube. We'd also see each other and get to talk at dinner whenever I did a workshop at the church, which has been almost every year. I was always struck by her smarts and funniness. It was clear she understood the *Course* much better than most people. Her background in psychology and her open-mindedness made her a natural, and I found her humor to be both inspired and entertaining.

If you're like me, you're going to enjoy this book, *The Top Ten Lies We Tell Ourselves—and How to Stop Living Them*. Dana has a gift for satire, and she's aware of the meaning of an important quotation from the *Course*, "Into eternity, where all is one [notice it doesn't say where all *was* one], there crept a tiny, mad idea, at which the Son of God remembered not to laugh. In his forgetting did the thought become a serious idea, and possible of both accomplishment and real effects. Together, we can laugh them both away, and understand that time cannot intrude upon eternity."

Although Dana has remembered to laugh, most people have forgotten to laugh at the silly dream-illusion known as the world. And that's a big part of the problem with the world. People take it so seriously, and they take their spirituality *very* seriously. And if there's one thing that Dr.

Dana realizes, it's that this world cannot be taken seriously. It's too crazy. In my first book, *The Disappearance of the Universe*, my teachers referred to this place we appear to find ourselves in as "psychoplanet." It's not worthy of our belief; only God is. So the *Course* also says, "Be vigilant only for God and His Kingdom."

That's why Dana isn't into the correction of others. The *Course* is very clear that mistakes should not be judged but overlooked instead. Most new students are not aware of that. In fact, you can usually tell if someone is a new student of ACIM. In the *Course*, our false identity that is based on separation is called "the ego." And that new student is usually very good at spotting the ego in somebody else. Yet there isn't anybody else—not really. So the *Course* speaks very precisely about judgment and the correction of error in your sisters and brothers: "The alertness of the ego to the errors of other egos is not the kind of vigilance the Holy Spirit would have you maintain."

Your real identity in the *Course* is perfect oneness, just like your Creator. God is represented in the *Course* by the Holy Spirit. Forgiveness—or the overlooking of the illusion of separation—is what is required if one is to achieve the goal of salvation, or enlightenment, in a reasonable instead of an unreasonable amount of time. As the *Course* so succinctly puts it, "A chief aim of the miracle worker is to save time." A miracle worker is anyone who practices forgiveness, coming from a place of cause and not effect. You don't forgive people because they've really done something; you forgive them because they haven't really done anything because this is your dream and you're the one who made them up in the first place. Dana's work is based on that knowledge, and her attitude is an all-forgiving one. I'm honored to be her friend, and I'm enthusiastic about recommending this book.

The best part of my experience of being an author and speaker for the last fifteen years has been the amazing people I've gotten to meet all over the world. Dana is a perfect example of that. I invite you to read this book with a sense of humor and an open attitude. The right part of your mind, where the Holy Spirit dwells, will thank you.

—Gary R. Renard, best-selling author of
*The Disappearance of the Universe, Your
Immortal Reality, Love Has Forgotten No
One,* and *The Lifetimes When Jesus and
Buddha Knew Each Other*

PREFACE

Depression has a taste—its bitterness will not leave your mouth no matter how many times you try to swallow it. Depression has a smell—its rancidness saturates every breath you inhale. Depression has a sound—its piercing shriek is so deafening that lips are moving all around you, but you can't make out a word. Depression has a look—its searing glare is reflected in eyes that only send daggers your way. Depression has a feel—its bone-chilling frost is like an anesthesia that never wears off.

Such was my reality for most of my first forty years. Few people around me knew the extent to which I was suffering, and that's exactly how I wanted it. I found it quite easy to act the exact opposite. Sure I felt like a fraud, but coming from a place of darkness doesn't necessarily birth insight. My hope is that in sharing my journey from all-encompassing self-hatred to all-encompassing love, you might be able to connect the dots quicker than I did or help someone you love do the same. You may want to grab a sweater as you read my story, which begins in Minnesota—known for its long winters, although it was my "mental" winter that seemed unending.

IT'S MY TRUTH AND I'M STICKING TO IT

I came home from school one day as a nine-year-old to find stacks of boxes in the kitchen and the smell of the woodstove burning in late spring. We were moving again— no big surprise, since we'd moved almost every year of my childhood. This time it was from the hills of Minnesota to the plains of North Dakota. We couldn't afford to take much with us, so it was the "nonessentials" of my own belongings I smelled burning in the woodstove, to lighten the load.

Such was a day in the life of my nomadic upbringing. My father clearly should have been born in another time period. Home to him was on the back of a horse, and he resisted taking roots or acquiring baggage. It was easy to identify him as the source of our family's chaos, resulting in my own unshakable gloom.

I was brought up Catholic, although I rarely enjoyed going to church or felt comfortable there. I held my religion at arm's length rather than embracing it, mainly because of the perceived effect it had on my mother. She attended

Catholic school and went to Mass daily. She told me that she remembers crying herself to sleep as a child because she was afraid she was having sinful thoughts that would send her to hell—perhaps the foundation for her struggle with depression. I'm sure the teenage pregnancy, of which I was the result, didn't help either. I thank her for presenting religion to me as a choice I could make, although there were no guarantees about escaping hell if I made the wrong one!

Dad was not a part of this conflict. His was alcoholism, which he struggled with since his teens, and my parents divorced, ironically enough, when he achieved sobriety. My mother became the primary caregiver of my much younger brother and sister, and I moved out on my own at seventeen. But my mother and I embarked on a parallel journey to find an end to the cycle of depression in our family. We both went into therapy and started college together, majoring in psychology.

Even though I always received top marks in school, I was far from a confident student. I had such social anxiety starting college that I remember eating lunch in the bathroom stall, so I wouldn't be seen as a loner sitting by myself in the common areas. By graduate school, I was having full-blown panic attacks. The only reason I didn't quit was I was even more terrified of the world outside the classroom. I chose to major in psychology because I thought that I could save myself from myself if I just learned the right theories of mind.

My relationships represented my distorted views about connection, founded on a childish decision never to be tricked by love. I could see that my parents weren't loving to each other long before they divorced. I always felt my father's love was conditional, while my mother loved me more than she loved herself, which didn't seem right either. This translated to my entering relationships in a detached way, very protective of myself. It was my belief that love would never be something I could count on. In my twenties, I had a series of relationships and even a short-lived marriage, where I tried to manufacture a sustainable feeling of love, to no avail.

MAKING MORE END RUNS AROUND FEAR

During this time, I focused on my career. Accomplishments gave me a sense of permanence. I was certain that once I earned a PhD, I would finally prove to myself and the world that I was smart, capable, and worthy. I received my doctorate from Purdue University and basked in that glory for about one month before fear and doubt slowly crept in again. I was working as a school psychologist, which enabled me to spend time with children—interactions I did enjoy, but I didn't feel I was really helping any of them.

It's clear that I had some awareness that I was being driven by fear, but I didn't know any other path to take.

My solution was to run away from it all, moving to the Los Angeles area with one of my girlfriends. I had been writing music after graduate school and performing with a local band. I always dreamed of being a pop star as a child, and now that I could support myself while trying to make it happen, it seemed slightly more realistic. At thirty, I met a producer with whom I felt a connection and started recording a demo. Meanwhile, I was partying alongside celebrities and other wannabes. This experience gave me an even more dysfunctional view of relationships. Now, instead of waiting to be attacked through rejection, I would be the one to attack first. My ego assured me this would guarantee my protection.

After a couple of years of this escapist indulgence, I still craved a true loving connection more than anything. I felt dead inside and knew I had to infuse myself with life if I was to truly thrive. It occurred to me that I could literally infuse myself with life by carrying a child. Maybe the experience of motherhood, the one role that I had yet to play, would finally connect me to unconditional love. When I met an exceedingly handsome man on Hermosa Beach, who wasn't a local, I was very motivated to make it work out, in part so I could run away yet again. After we spent just five weekends together over a six-month period, I left my LA life behind and moved to the other coast. We were married the following year and had our son the year after that.

Motherhood, however, did not bring about the transformative experience of love I was hoping for. Somehow, the act of bringing life into the world simultaneously drained what was left out of mine. It was important to me to be a stay-at-home mom, but I always defined my worth outside of myself, by my accomplishments. My depression was compounded by my perceived loss of identity through my profession and by the loss of my dream of becoming a famous singer-songwriter. As I was living through the ego, where internal fear is projected outward, the message my newborn son reflected back to me was that I was failing at the one task I had given myself. He had severe food allergies and feeding issues from birth (eosinophilic esophagitis) and was far from content. I hadn't fully recovered from the first round of postpartum depression I experienced with him when I got pregnant with my daughter, which seemed to compound the effect. My lowest moments were waiting for me after her birth, which finally and thankfully led me to reach a point of surrender.

A FAINT CRY FOR HELP

My ego had run a long campaign, mostly victorious, to convince me that I was worthy only of punishment. I already felt dead inside, but now I was at risk for making it official. Instead of taking that step, I made a faint, almost undetectable cry for help in my mind. I said it in jest, almost like a challenge: *If there is a higher power, which there probably isn't, then come and save me. But you probably won't. You'll have to do all the work since I'm not in a position to extend myself to you.*

That is exactly what happened though. That small opening created space for my self-evolution to occur. It wasn't instantaneous but rather a gradual removal of the layers of fear over the course of several years—and it's still happening. Mine has been a journey from anguish and steadfast despair to joy and steadfast hope. And I continue to use joy as my compass.

INTRODUCTION

If laughter is the best medicine for physical illness, what might it do for our spiritual ailments? Having been on the spiritual path for a while now, I've found that my barometer for whether or not I'm progressing is laughter. If I can't find the humor in a faulty belief I've uncovered, I'm probably not ready to let it go. After all, the path to enlightenment requires letting go of all the "enheavyment" we've built up. We just can't take our little selves and the world too seriously, for they contradict the True Self we share equally with God beyond this world. (Just wait—I'll get to that.)

For me, this realization originated from the inspirational text A *Course in Miracles* (ACIM), which presents a psychological/spiritual thought system based on forgiveness and changing our basic motivation from fear to love. Perhaps that sounds like a mouthful to you. It did to me at first too. In fact, I sincerely wish I'd chosen a spiritual path that I could talk about while still appearing to be normal, but that horse escaped the barn a while ago and hasn't been seen since.

Over two-and-a-half million copies of the *Course* have been sold worldwide since its release four decades ago. Many teachers of the *Course* have emerged, and I feel called to join them. Not because the masses are in need of a conversion, but because the *Course* reminds us that we all learn what we teach—and I could still use some help seeing past my own massive illusions. Since our minds are joined, each of us individually can affect the whole. My mentor, Gary Renard, set a great example for how to share the depth of the *Course* with lightness and humor, despite some reservations. In his first book, *The Disappearance of the Universe*, he wrote, "If I told people that God didn't create the world, I have a feeling it would probably go over about as big as a fart in the elevator."

A NEW FOUNDATION

My existence—pre-*Course*—was built on a crumbling foundation of fear. Upon the recommendation of a trusted colleague, I started reading the *Course* and got my first glimpse at what a solid foundation of love might feel like. I remember the first time I held the *Course* in my hand and literally felt it vibrate. I somehow knew I'd begun an epic journey. Yet there is no magic in the book itself. In fact, the *Course* invites us to reflect on its principles and then forget them. It advocates holding onto nothing, even the teaching itself. The problem is that we are unaware of all the ways in which we are tightly gripping our fears, clouding our awareness of love as our true identity. And that means telling ourselves a bunch of lies—of which this book reveals only the top ten!

And now for a spoiler alert. All ten ego-generated "lies" discussed herein can be corrected by understanding the one illusion that is the epicenter of all self-deceptions: the "tiny, mad idea"[1] that it's possible to be separate from our Source and from each other. According to A *Course in Miracles*, this twisted idea gave birth to the ego, the mistaken identity we all know and love so well.

It's imperative to understand the distinction between our *little self* and its faulty attempt to be the source of its own creations and our *True Self*, which is permanently linked to the actual Source of all creation. We decide which identity badge to wear in any given moment. The choice is ours to make.

Our ego identity or *little self* is . . .		Our Spirit identity or *True Self* is . . .
Rooted in fear	→	Love
Confined to a body	→	Vast
Convinced it is perishable	→	Infinite
The experience of individuality	→	Oneness
Conflict seeking	→	Peace
Focused on scarcity	→	Abundance
Suspicious by nature	→	Trust
Fixated on judgment	→	Acceptance
Fueled by grandiosity	→	Grandeur
On a mission to condemn	→	Innocence
Loyal to no one, not even you	→	Faith
Withholding by nature	→	Extension
Fumbling in the dark	→	Light
Constantly seeking answers	→	Knowledge
Trapped within illusion	→	Reality
In a state of flux at all times	→	Constant
The denial of miracles	→	Divine
Our personal and collective hell	→	Heaven

There seems to be a clear winner. Right? Together, we'll explore why the ego is so tricky to let go of and also why we must. The ego, or fear-soaked part of our minds, is happiest when we listen to it intently and try to do everything it asks, even when it makes no sense. Our spiritual growth also depends on listening to the ego intently, but only so we can learn how *not* to do what it asks. This book is about looking and laughing at the hidden and often quite shocking messages of the ego that we tend to accept as truth without question.

SETTING AN INTENTION

I recommend a gentle, lighthearted "roasting" of our self-deceptions over time in order to avoid nasty ego backlash, which is really our own deep-seated belief that we don't deserve to feel better. Miracles usually come in small incremental packages, but each one is worth opening. In fact that's what time is for: the gradual unlearning of our self-destruct mode (engineered by the ego) in favor of a healing mode (led by Spirit, which is awareness that our true identity of shared perfection could never be altered).

Each of the top ten "lies" comes with a twenty-four-hour challenge. Therefore, it takes a minimum of only ten days to complete this book for maximum benefit. Such a deal! But if the challenges are ignored, I reserve the right to blame readers for any lack of results . . . which is a nice segue to the first lie on the list: *Nothing is more important than being right!*

THE TOP TEN LIES WE TELL OURSELVES

LIE #10

NOTHING IS MORE IMPORTANT THAN BEING RIGHT

(and, of course,
you always are)

Most likely, your first reaction to hearing this lie is, "*Boy, do* I *know someone who believes that!*" If we are being honest with ourselves, though, we all have a knee-jerk reaction to find the jerk "out there" who's responsible for any given problem before a finger can possibly be pointed at ourselves. Many times, we automatically look outward for the source of the problem when it comes to assigning blame.

This is because we unknowingly suffer from the worldwide epidemic of "directionality confusion." In other words, we have to learn that nothing is coming *at* us, mandating our immediate judgment and response. In fact, it's all coming *from* us—although we would certainly rather not accept this as the way things are.

What appears to be happening is that there are thousands upon thousands (a reliable, endless supply) of faulty, wrong-thinking human beings around us—from willful, mind-blowing idiots all the way down to those hapless, good-natured people who just don't know any better. All these people are regularly saying or doing things that we can easily judge as clearly wrong. Thus we join the endless crusade of the ego: to elevate each of us personally as the gold standard of all that's right and sensible. Of course, that requires constant vigilance in order to keep seeing who is in the wrong and point them out for everyone's benefit.

But what if everything is actually happening in the other direction? We can't entirely suppress the ego's hidden anxiety, which is that—for each of us—**I'm the one who is wrong about everything**. Specifically, I was profoundly wrong that separating from my Source would be an improvement on perfection. Since I unconsciously fear being punished for this mindless choice, I must invent an "other" who is wrong, so I can pretend I am right. To make it more convincing, I'll make up countless millions of others who are wrong about this or that, and I'll make up just a few choice others who mostly agree with me. Thus the battle lines are drawn. It's guaranteed that I'll always be outnumbered, so I can feel persecuted, perhaps even leading to my eventual martyrdom. To make all this even more convincing, I'll choose to forget I made up the whole mess.

LET'S ANALYZE
(lying on a couch is optional)

Classical psychology can shed some light on this budding awareness. Anna Freud was Sigmund's youngest child of six. Her father was the first to articulate that whatever we suppress in ourselves we *project* onto others. Anna took it a step further with the idea of *reaction formation*—that is, when a person avoids one position (being wrong) by insisting the opposite is true (being right).

We can use this concept to measure our resistance to change and growth. The greater the certainty we feel that we're right about anything in particular, the greater our unwillingness to acknowledge that we are actually wrong about *everything*. In her book *The Ego and the Mechanisms of Defense*, Anna explained that "indications of obsessional exaggeration suggest that it is of the nature of a reaction (formation) and that it conceals a long-standing conflict." Additionally, this human tendency acts as a form of "permanent protection." This means that we cover our tracks well, or at least we think we have. However, both the *Course* and the Freuds are happy to point out that what we deny inside is clearly visible outside. We only need look at our perception of the world to have a perfect view of this hidden conflict in action. To the extent I believe what needs changing is out in the world or external, I can pretend it's not within me.

But denial has its perks: we get to be God . . . or sort of. That is, we choose to live in a massive illusion that we're projecting at every moment and calling it "reality."

THE (BLAME) GAME OF LIFE

The *Course* asks us, "Do you prefer that you be right or happy?"[1] The answer depends on who you want to hang out with. If the ego is your constant companion, being right makes you happy, but that kind of happiness depends on identifying who is wrong. The ego can show you just how effortless that task is and how big the reward: *never having to look at your own part in your troubles.*

If Spirit is your guide, though, admitting the wrongness of everything the ego has been telling you is the path to lasting happiness. Spirit will gently correct your error in thinking and, once corrected, your natural flow of happiness will emerge. Happiness can even become your new normal, for it's something you actually already possess in abundance.

A required first step is to look deeply at our unconscious need to assign blame. Frankly, I've noticed that it feels good to make at least ten people wrong before my morning tea! Watching the news as soon as I wake up speeds up this process considerably, so turning on the box full of idiots is so helpful when I'm in a hurry. Otherwise, the cast of characters in my own house will do fine for starters. Assigning blame is like the gravitational pull holding us securely in this made-up world. But when we stop blaming, we can literally float above this world like an astronaut in training.

Let's continue our experiment with weightlessness. I invite you to lose your "self" and find your "Self" in this chart, starting with our default setting and working up to our final destination—a complete and total shift in perception of wrong vs. right.

THE BLAME CONTINUUM
Where Are You?

1. Hand cramps from all of the *finger pointing* at the world	*"It's not complicated. You are obviously wrong!"*
2. Slightly hesitant *finger pointing* at the world	*"It's a little tricky, but who am I kidding? I'm probably right."*
3. *Finger pointing* at the world *and* self	*"Your hands are just as dirty as mine. Who really knows who's at fault?"*
4. *Finger pointing* directed *only* at self	*"I see the pattern now. I've needed you to be wrong over and over again."*
5. No *finger pointing*, too busy holding stomach in laughter	*"It's not complicated. I am playing both sides and making it all up!"*

1. "It's not complicated. You are obviously wrong!" This phase affords us a sense of superficial peace. There is considerable unrest below the surface, but it gets blown off with regularity, just like the geyser Old Faithful.

The release of this unconscious pressure—in the form of spouting out accusations—is an irresistible attraction. And our accusations are always justified—we make sure of that by inventing a stupid world that constantly needs our corrections! Here, the ego reigns supreme without question. And the world of bodies is "proof of life" in this phase. Of course we are separate bodies with separate interests, separate wills, and separate destinies, fighting amongst ourselves for control of the whole mess. Only a New Age crazy would think otherwise. Right?

2. **"It's a little tricky, but who am I kidding? I'm probably right."** Here we've taken a small but monumental step in the right direction. It implies a slight willingness to be wrong, even if it is limited to a particular situation for a fleeting moment. Although the ego allows the possibility of taking some responsibility for wrongness, the "other" is by no means off the hook. However, this shift in thinking *is* a start worth recognizing.

3. **"Your hands are just as dirty as mine. Who really knows who's at fault?"** Still guided primarily by the ego, this kind of uncertainty is yet focused on the external, made-up world—the realm of endless problems and no solutions. The willingness to no longer view ourselves as blameless in the whole mess is of great significance. However, insufficient trust has been established in the "other way" to stay with it long enough to reap the rewards.

It can actually feel like you're joining with others here, but the attitude of "I'm *a lowlife; you're a lowlife. Cheers!*" is no way to reach the high life.

4. "**I see the pattern now. I've needed you to be wrong over and over again**." This is a fragile but empowering phase. It is terrifying to release all others as recipients of blame, for the weight of the world now rests singly on our own shoulders. It's precisely here, though, that we get a first glimpse at our limitless power that we have misused and denied. What if we could fix it *all* for ourselves and everyone? Would we do it if we were shown exactly how?

5. "**It's not complicated. I am playing both sides and making the whole thing up!**" Finally, a triumph over the ego. The faulty idea that we could be separate from each other and our Source despite "evidence" in the world is now discredited under the proper framework. There is no longer a fear-based payoff to avoid self-punishment by making the "other" wrong, because it is understood that there is no "other." Personally, you are not to blame either, for there is no personal version of you. We are all released from blame together. We are truly at peace, for we are secure in our identification with our inherent oneness.

We must be gentle and patient with ourselves in this process. We can't go from the bottom of the chart to the top in an instant. Well, we could actually, but our resistance to healing is usually too strong for that to occur. It takes time, but that's what time is for when used correctly—for healing instead of hiding in blame and shame.

CAN I GET A WITNESS?

The *Course* tells us that "the world you see is but the idle witness that you were right."[2] Our world is idle because nothing is really happening here that has any effect on eternity. The word *witness* is used since we are watching this nonsense—and only watching, even though we think we're intimately involved. The reference to "you were right" is written in past tense because we see only the past. It's over, and we'll experience all conflict as over when we're ready to give it up. We must feel safe enough to do so. But since we are almost always secretly thinking that something catastrophic already happened, and will keep happening because of what we think we did, the smoke screen is hard to see through.

There will come a time when we realize that we've been watching a dark and sinister, poorly written rerun, with a shockingly **happy** ending! Stock up on popcorn while you can.

IT'S AN EXERCISE
(mental stretching required)

Find a moment to connect with your thoughts. You don't have to be sitting in full lotus with your favorite scented candle burning. The physical environment will never ensure our peace of mind because we didn't set up the world that way. So however you choose to center yourself in the midst of our constant chaos, find the tiniest bit of space in your mind and use it. Ask yourself these two important questions:

1. *Who have I locked up in a penitentiary for the eternally "wrong"?*
2. *What judge do I consult to confirm my sentencing of others?*

My answers to these questions always reflect what I don't want to face in myself at any given moment, that someone else must be wrong for me to feel right. And since that "release" of tension is short-lived, it only makes sense that I have a vast pool of options to serve as the accused. I've come to realize that whether I do the accusing myself or witness other's accusations, it has a similar effect of appeasing my little self at the expense of remembering my True Self.

When I worked in an office setting and was feeling underappreciated, I'd have lunch with colleagues who were certain to bash the boss along with me. Or, even better, I'd let someone else rant and say nothing, nodding my head in agreement while thinking that I was better than the person ranting. It felt so good to have someone else to do the dirty work for me!

If my kids are breaking me down, I call on a girlfriend to talk about bad parenting choices of our mutual friends or bad parents who make headlines. Maybe that's why my children act out right next to me, which is so "wrong," but at least I don't have to do the kicking and screaming myself. I get to remain the peacemaker while still unknowingly enjoying the fighting vicariously.

When my security feels threatened—like when we recently relocated our family—nothing does the trick like reopening childhood wounds. I'll call my sister, Lisa, to talk about all the things our parents didn't do to help us feel secure. We know that script of timeworn complaints very well, and we can efficiently get right to it when we need to. It's so nice to be of assistance to each other in this ruse!

As for my husband, forget it! I try to be subtle about it, but generally he serves as my reliable wellspring of wrongness. I use him like a cell phone that needs a daily boost on the charger. It's not that I complain out loud. In fact I rarely share the list of all the ways he is wrong. I keep it private for my own personal enjoyment, although it feels more like compulsive necessity than enjoyment, if I'm being honest.

THE VOLCANO WITHIN

These questionable habits remind me of the famous line from the movie *Knotting Hill*. Instead of Julia Roberts poignantly saying, "I'm just a girl, standing in front of a boy, asking him to love me," I'm more like, "I'm just a girl, sitting on top of a volcano, trying to keep it from blowing my judgmental hatred everywhere and burning you all alive." What I've learned from my daily interactions with others is that lurking underneath the most minor irritation is a raging inferno.

Looking beyond our inner circles of family, friends, and colleagues, we can use strangers, foreigners, and crazy people in the news in the same way. It's simple sport to blame and judge other people, plucking their faults off the blame tree like they are low-hanging fruit. But we all harbor murderous thoughts and can find them if we look deeply enough.

I used to follow the common instinct that says, "Don't look!" That didn't really work, though, and that's why I was crippled with depression for most of my first forty years. The good news is there is another way. It's dependent on our willingness to look at the darkness—the big picture of how we've been mistaken about everything, including our own identity—but not alone. The light of Spirit can guide us through it.

IT'S A LIFE-OR-DEATH MATTER

"Are thoughts, then, dangerous?" asks the *Course*, and answers: "To bodies, yes!"[3] However, the *Course* also makes it clear that never, even for an instant, have we ever been in a body. Dr. Kenneth Wapnick expanded on the danger of thoughts in his book *Journey through the Text of A Course in Miracles*: "We have judgmental thoughts and suddenly feel them in our bodies and become ill, or think we have hurt others who in retaliation will cause us pain and upset." He goes on to quote the *Course* as follows: "The thoughts that seem to kill are those that teach the thinker that he *can* be killed. And so he 'dies' because of what he learned."[4]

It was our own decision then, for the illusion of vulnerability that effectively denied our changeless invulnerability. Yet this predicament can be reversed merely by acknowledging it. We can recognize that we are immortal right now, not at some point in the future if we're deemed worthy!

It follows then that we've been "wrong" about death. It's a concept contrived from nothing, and to nothing it shall return when we no longer have a purpose for it: as an imagined punishment for the false sin of destroying perfect oneness. Death does not represent a natural process, a random event, a punishment, an escape, or any change at all. We made a decision to be in this world, which we could do only by becoming a dream figure. But, in fact, we are not of this world. Our Source of love is unaware and unaffected by our collective dream of what love's opposite looks, feels, and smells like. Just like a sleeping dream that can seem so very real, we will awaken from it entirely and understand its complete and total unreality.

Until then, we no longer need concern ourselves with who is being punished enough in the dream. This dream is an equal opportunity punisher. Justice will not prevail because the dream itself is an injustice. There is no natural order, only natural disorder. Even if things appear to be going your way and you momentarily attain near-perfection in body, status, or even love, it's all on the way out. Nothing impermanent is real. We are afraid to acknowledge all this because it sounds like extreme pessimism. Yet what lies just beyond extreme pessimism—nothing will ever be right—is permanent optimism or our remembrance that all is right. It can be no other way except in a dream.

A COMEDY OF ERRORS

I was sitting in meditation right before going to bed one night, which I usually do for five minutes or so. It happened to be a few days after the passing of actor and comedian Robin Williams. I was always a fan of his work; I remember showing the entire *Dead Poets Society* movie to my "Intro to Educational Psychology" class the first semester I taught it as a grad student. But that was mainly because I really didn't know what I was doing or how to fill the time. As I began thinking of Robin, his apparent suffering as well as my own, I got the feeling he had a message for me, reinforcing how we had it all wrong and even laughing at the idea of it. In my mind, we had a conversation:

"What do you want to tell me?" I asked.

"Will you help people understand depression?" he replied.

"Yes," I agreed, "but only if you help me make it funny."

"Of course!"

After that "agreement," I felt my whole body tingle, like a supercaffeinated college freshman. I went to bed as I had planned on doing, but my eyes were wide open and my thoughts were racing. What was coming to me, rapid-fire, were ideas for a comedic, educational program about depression in the form of a one-woman show on Broadway—filled with elaborate props, skits, and songs. After an hour or so of downloading, I told Robin that this was all great stuff, but I really needed to sleep right now. Instantly, the tingling and rush of ideas stopped.

I laughed at the immediate response to my request and went to sleep. I have yet to perform on Broadway, but I did turn the experience into a YouTube video series called *Did You Forget to Laugh?* By the way, I don't believe I was "chosen" as a special recipient of the brilliance of Robin Williams. I believe we all have access to anyone, from all time periods, all of the time. That's the cool thing about oneness. We can't escape each other even if we wanted to!

We have overlearned who we mistakenly thought we were, but guidance comes in many forms, as a constant reminder of what we really are. Ultimately, though, each of us is our own guru. It only takes one of us to restore sanity to all of us, and that person is *you*!—No pressure! Should you choose to accept this mission—and you already have—you will be met with all the guidance you need to succeed.

MIRROR, MIRROR ON THE WALL

Who is the most horrible person of all? I certainly am—if all I am is a body that's closer to dying every day while holding on to "private" but projected thoughts of hatred directed at everyone and everything. We all are like this when we think with the ego. And we know by now how desperately the ego wants to be right about everything.

I remember when I first announced to people that I was majoring in psychology. To my surprise, I saw a look of sheer panic on the faces of some of the most well-adjusted people I knew. Perhaps they worried I would someday have access to the private thoughts that they obviously were ashamed to acknowledge.

It's like baking cookies with lemon juice instead of sugar . . . no, wait, that actually sounds good. You know what I mean. The sourness would be part of the cookies, just like it's baked into the world. We can't change the recipe to something tastier, because we only used crappy ingredients. We'd all like to pretend that we are the one who holds the sugar, but none of us are. We can adjust to the bad taste, as we have, or just stop eating—making sweetness and goodness objects of desire.

CONQUERING THE LIE

The way to escape from the endless loop of playing judge and jury with ourselves is to stop taking new cases in the courtroom. To wrap up all existing cases, refrain from focusing on the specifics of a case, and shift to a more general analysis. Each case seems unique when viewed under the ego's microscope, where different players and different circumstances emerge. With Spirit's vision, we understand that all of our court cases are exactly the same. We can throw them all out simultaneously. Thankfully, we don't have to search for truth because truth is what we are. We are only called to deny what is false—the idea that we could be separate from each other and our Source even if we wanted to be, which we don't!

Healing, then, is one-size-fits-all. With the ego's thought system, we're completely unaware that we're wrong about everything, all the time, without exception. While we suspect that something has gone terribly wrong, we're pretty certain it must be someone else's fault. Following guidance from Spirit, we become aware of our ridiculously magnificent error; it's all very black and white. The ego wants us to search for fifty thousand shades of gray so that we're constantly preoccupied with the analysis and judgment of others. But since there is only one of us here appearing as many, all judgment is self-judgment. And when all judgment is set aside, the True Self you could never destroy shines through with the greatest of ease.

TAKE THE CHALLENGE AND BE THE CHANGE

Starting on the path of change only requires a little willingness from you to see things differently. Let's start here with our first twenty-four-hour challenge: **For today and today only, I am willing to believe I might be wrong about absolutely everything.**

To inspire you, here's a sampling from my list of errors just today:

- I thought my ham-and-almond-cheese omelet had around eight grams of fat, but it was closer to twelve. (EFFECT ON REALITY = NONE)

- I thought I knew my real parents, but they are my dream-figure parents. (EFFECT ON REALITY = NONE)

- I thought I had more cat litter, but I must have forgotten to buy it. (EFFECT ON REALITY = NONE)

- I thought my body was real when I got called back a second time for a mammogram to investigate irregular tissue, but now I remember that it's not. (EFFECT ON REALITY = NONE)

Try it on now, for your own twenty-four-hour challenge: **For today and today only, I am willing to believe I might be wrong about absolutely everything.** You may be shocked at just how error-prone you can be!

LIE
#9

THERE IS NOT ENOUGH OF ANYTHING TO GO AROUND

(so take your share by
any means possible)

Simply watching the news is all that's required to see this lie in action. However, the ego's belief in scarcity plays out in our daily offscreen lives as well, in both blatantly obvious and extremely subtle ways that are worth some serious looking into. If we're lucky, the investigation will yield some comic relief from an otherwise dire situation. It all comes down to our deep-seated fear of emptiness within. Instead of looking at this fear to evaluate if it's justified, we tend to let it "**FESTER**": We Fear Emptiness So we Try to Evict Reason.

DOWN THE RABBIT HOLE OF SCARCITY

The ego operates from an either/or mentality. Either you have something of value or I do, but we can never have it at the same time. Following this message down the ego's rabbit hole, we'll discover something else: we secretly believe that whatever you have was stolen from me and I deeply resent you for it. But wait! Beneath that resentment is the fear that I *actually stole from you and ultimately from my*

Source! Since I deserve to be punished for stealing—not to mention falsely accusing you *and* God—I keep re-creating a world of scarcity that constantly threatens my very life.

This is painfully circular thinking, of course, but the ego would rather we don't look too closely at that. Spirit's correction for this ridiculous predicament is a thought of oneness: we heal "together or not at all."[1] Since our separation from each other is just an illusion, *each* of us can effect change for the *whole* of us. We need only accept that we deserve to get out of the hell we've made. The ego will keep inviting us back to its dangerous playground— the world—which seems to contain exactly what we want. Somehow, though, it's always just out of reach. Our error is in repeatedly following this fleeting fancy, placing value on the valueless. The "valueless" is anything that can change, and anything that can change will never fill the void created by believing in our separation from Source.

THE HOARDER WITHIN

Let's take the example of a compulsive hoarder, who collects vast amounts of possessions and demonstrates extreme anxiety at the thought of parting with them, even at the cost of adverse effects on one's health, finances, and relationships. From a *Course* perspective, this behavior is symbolic of an "outside picture of an inward condition."[2]

It reflects the ego's warning that resources always run out, and it's wise to prepare for this impending loss ahead of time. The addiction derives from a panicky feeling that even a highly focused preparedness may not be enough protection.

Most of us do not meet the clinical definition of a hoarder, but subtler forms of hoarding are just as harmful. (I'm not talking about my hiding place in the kitchen for gourmet potato chips and fancy candy that I don't want to share. That's just healthy self-love.) I've only recently become aware of my own mental hoarding behaviors. For example, I catch myself hoarding what I consider to be good ideas for my self-help social-media posts. I have pages of them, but fear that if I share them all, I'll be left with a blank page. Surely there can't be an unlimited supply of good ideas!

I've learned, though, that when I force myself to share everything I have, I restore a natural flow of well-being. Holding on to anything, even a good idea, blocks this flow. I find success and sweetness when I hold on to nothing.

LET'S ANALYZE
(lying on a couch is optional)

Insight can be gained by looking at Abraham Maslow's "Hierarchy of Needs," a psychological theory of human motivation. He makes a distinction between basic-level needs, such as survival, security, and love/belonging, and higher-level needs of self-esteem and self-actualization. Maslow concluded that if basic-level needs are not met, anxiety will prevent us from going any further. And, in fact, the ego's goal is for us to flatline near the bottom in perpetuity, as desperate scavengers in a dark, desolate world. By contrast, Spirit teaches us that through consistent denial of the false, we will experience the changeless Truth about ourselves. And the changeless Truth is that ultimately we have no needs. We are completely provided for by our eternal Source of abundance in every way possible.

Interestingly, Maslow fashioned a peak for his pyramid called "self-transcendence," topping off his theory with a spiritual vibe. In his book *Toward a Psychology of Being*, he revealed the essence of this high point, which embodies our ultimate conflict: "It is precisely the godlike in ourselves that we are ambivalent about, fascinated by and fearful of, motivated to and defensive against." This line of thinking is congruent with the *Course*. We are "simultaneously worms and gods," says Maslow. Our choice, then, is to value our separate will and illusive individuality—as a worm among worms—or value our shared will and collective existence as equal to God. Separately we are nothing, and together we are everything—quite literally!

IT'S AN EXERCISE
(mental stretching required)

Trusting the naturally abundant flow of life can be terrifying. The ego is quick to sort through your memories for evidence of when you chose to "let go" and it all went wrong, casting a shadow of impending gloom over your future. Let's resist that habit by finding the natural flow of abundance.

You will need a blank piece of paper, drawn into four quadrants. We'll start with examining our attachments to possessions, as a precursor to the deeper issue. Fill in at least three entries in each quadrant fitting the descriptions in the chart.

MATERIAL THINGS
(The Easier Part)

LOATHE 'em . . . *Just haven't gotten around to throwing it all out.*	*INDIFFERENT* about 'em . . . *Don't really care enough to go through it all.*
1. _____	1. _____
2. _____	2. _____
3. _____	3. _____

ATTACHED to 'em . . . I'd keep this stuff unless the house was on fire. Then forget it.	TREASURE 'em . . . I'd be strongly tempted to run back into the burning house for this stuff!
1. _____	1. _____
2. _____	2. _____
3. _____	3. _____

A sampling from my list includes:

- jeans that fit only after a bad stomach bug (LOATHE);
- high school yearbooks (INDIFFERENT);
- 1980s music collection (ATTACHED); and
- a couple of pieces of jewelry (TREASURE).

Of course we need certain possessions for survival, and there is nothing wrong with preferring to have other material things as well. The stumbling block occurs when our identity is tied to particular items, usually in the form of providing a false sense of worthiness or status.

We all have an inkling that nothing impermanent exists in the grand scheme of things, so let's dig even deeper. Using a new sheet of paper drawn into four quadrants, fill in each square with three key past experiences. Set the intention of honestly reviewing your best and worst moments.

PAST EXPERIENCES
(The Harder Part)

LOATHE it . . . Would love to forget it ever happened.	INDIFFERENT about it . . . Don't really care enough to wish there'd been a different outcome.
1. _____ 2. _____ 3. _____	1. _____ 2. _____ 3. _____
ATTACHED to it . . . I love keeping this memory around. What's the harm?	TREASURE it . . . You won't be able to pry this memory loose from my cold, dead brain.
1. _____ 2. _____ 3. _____	1. _____ 2. _____ 3. _____

The memory I **LOATHE** is my early attempt to shut out my stepmother, which culminated in a written manifesto about why we should just accept that it was never going to work out between us and that it would be best if we didn't see each other apart from weddings and funerals. No shortage of drama there! What a difference twenty years can make though. I've learned to stop focusing on what she was seemingly taking from me, and shifting to an awareness of what she is giving me—peace of mind that my father is taken care of by someone who adores him.

My **INDIFFERENT** memory—now good for a laugh—is when I somehow made it on to a semiprofessional in-line skate racing team, only to fall on my ass within seconds of my first race.

My **ATTACHED** moment is when my grandmother admitted to me that I was her favorite. (Ah, that's still like a cup of hot cocoa on a cold day.) And my **TREASURE** moment is my daughter telling me that I'm the best mom *ever* (which cancels out at least three screams of "I hate you!" that came earlier).

Next, review your list of past experiences and note how similar your emotional responses are within each quadrant or box, and how different they are across quadrants—ranging from negative, to neutral, to positive. Spirit is asking us to override our urge to judge and sort our experiences differently in the made-up world, instead bundling them together as *all the same*. Pick one entry from each category and apply this by saying: "This *Loathe it* memory is the same as one under *Attached to it*. This *Indifferent about it* moment is the same as one under *Treasure it*."

Ego-driven experiences all have the intent of helping us hide out in this world, thus delaying our ultimate healing. The ego secretly urges you to hang on to your *Loathe it* list because it reveals your "true colors," meaning that you deserve to suffer for what you've done. Spirit—the memory of our true identity as perfect love—does nothing more than shine light on this hidden agenda, so that we are able to choose against it. This seems to engender a battle between fear and love, although that's entirely our imagining. A battle requires two actual opponents—but only love is real.

THE GIVING VS. RECEIVING MYTH

With the ego as our guide, giving and receiving are viewed as two separate processes. This belief brings on an inner tug-of-war. A considerable amount of effort is expended just to keep ourselves standing upright, holding on to our fair share of things. We may fear that if we loosen our grip for even an instant, the inevitable result will be a face full of mud.

Spirit can help us reinterpret the game with the knowledge that there is only One of us here appearing as many. What we give, we receive simultaneously. The tug-of-war rope becomes a circle, with you holding both ends.

Within the dream world we share, we can't really give anything, because there isn't anything here—including us. Since we do experience the world and our separate bodies as real, the *Course* meets us where (we think) we are: "Miracles are healing because they supply a lack; they are performed by those who temporarily have more for those who temporarily have less."[3] When we give, then, we demonstrate to ourselves that we have enough. From there we can go on to recognize that giving is our natural state, and it's all we can really do. Only in the illusion does taking seem like not only a viable option, but an absolute necessity.

GIVING TO GET WHAT ISN'T THERE

We've established that giving without reservation is the path to the truth about ourselves. Let's contrast that path with how the ego goes about "giving." The ego *gives to get*, since it's constantly evaluating itself in relation to other egos and preoccupied with the myth of scarcity.

This doesn't mean that we are called to give away all of our possessions, titles, and relationships in order to prove that we're spiritual. Sacrifice plays no part in spiritual growth—quite the opposite, actually. Spirit is only asking us to look closely at what we do, and how it feels, when we blindly follow the ego through a maze of dark tunnels leading nowhere. Ultimately we will decide we no longer want to do that. We don't lose anything in this process except our incorrect perceptions.

For example, my role as a mother is one that I obsess over more than any other. Of course I don't want to ruin my little gifts from God! Is that what they really are though? Or was the image of them generated from the same fear machine that I—as a separate individual—came from? Spirit tells me I can't screw up what doesn't exist, unless I want to believe that I can, as a form of self-punishment for having chosen my separateness in the first place.

The possibility that my kids aren't real seemed not only insane, initially, but the ultimate disappointment to a mother's ego. Ultimately, though, this belief led not to passive resignation but to impassioned action instead. I'm much closer to consistently responding to them with the love that I *am*, not the love I'm waiting to receive before I ration it out carefully. In other words, I'm no longer using them to fill a void in myself . . . on a good day anyway.

THE BOTTOMLESS PIT OF LACK

The world we see is an *effect* of the bottomless pit of lack within and not the *cause*. The cause was our choice to invest in it and swear by its existence with our illusory lives. Of course, we'd prefer to see the problem as outside ourselves, even if this means playing the victim of injustices great and small. The world can be no other way, when the habit of hiding still has something to offer us.

To bring it closer to home, let's take a look at our own personal hideouts—our bodies. In the book *Form versus Content*, philosopher Ken Wapnick wrote, "The body was made to be an instrument of scarcity. If I do not fill my lungs with oxygen, my body with food and water, and my psychological body with love and attention, something terrible will surely happen."

The ego's hidden message is that we must stay focused on our bodies and the world, which are clearly in need of our constant vigilance. When we believe this hidden message, we forget that we chose this paradigm for ourselves and everyone all at once. Yet we *can* change our mind, saving ourselves and everyone all at once, at any point in time. This would actually mark the *end* of time— our departure from the dream world to the eternal reality we never really left.

Does that sound amazing or terrifying? I would say a mixture of both, if I'm being honest.

A NEW VANTAGE POINT

What a beautiful release it can be to remember that we are dreaming—and only dreaming—all the time! This knowledge is not an escape or a new place to hide, but rather an entrance to a deeper awareness. It's a new lens by which to look at reality. It allows us to see the *symbolic* value in everything—for that is the only value it has, and even that value is temporary.

The *Course* makes no distinction between sleeping and waking dreams, clarifying that they are equally unreal. However, we are more willing to see events in our sleeping dreams as merely symbols, without judgment or attachment. While awake, it would also serve us well to view all events as symbols—of hiding or healing. Typically, though, we struggle to make sense of everything that happens as the "real" stories of our lives.

I've been fascinated with dreams since I was a child and have often kept a dream journal. When I read in the *Course* that we're meant to turn over all of our experiences to Spirit for reinterpretation, I thought it would be to my advantage to include my dream life. Internally I asked, "Spirit, if I'm not getting a lesson you're trying to teach me while I'm awake, you can try to sneak it in while I'm asleep."

Shortly after setting that intention, I had what I would describe as an *out-of-body* dream. In it, I was watching myself and other bodies from above. At first I was enjoying the vantage point of a 360-degree view of myself while walking along a crowded street. I was thinking, "I guess my butt doesn't look too big in those shorts." And "my shoulders are rounded. I really need to stand up straighter." Then I thought, "Why do I think I'm *that* body and not any of the others?" The answer: *"You can learn the most from that one."*

Analyzing this dream the next morning, I recognized that the first critical voice I heard was clearly the judgmental ego. The question of "Why this body and not the others?" came from my free will to choose which teacher to follow. The answer of "Stay with it. You have more to learn from that body" came from the gentleness of Spirit.

From this dream, I also realized that I felt more anchored, protected, and safe than ever before. I knew that if the scene I was watching—my body and others walking down a busy street—no longer existed, then I would go on completely unscathed. Even though I woke up to "a dry and dusty world, where starved and thirsty creatures come to die,"[4] as the *Course* brazenly puts it, I don't feel as starved, or thirsty, or worried about my impending death as I used to be. And that's a gift of peace that not even Amazon can deliver.

MOVING OUT OF "SCARE-CITY"

Our spiritual goal is to understand that our true Source of abundance is beyond the image of scarcity we made in its place. Because we are unknowingly so invested in the idea of scarcity, we're going to continue watching ourselves manipulate others to get what we want overtly (like a tyrant), covertly (like a martyr), or any way in between from moment to moment. When we do it with the ego, then it's really happening and reflects the "worm" that we are. When we do it with Spirit, we can remember that it's not really happening and could never represent who we really are. It's just a temporary case of mistaken identity with no consequences whatsoever in reality. This may sound like we're letting ourselves off the hook, but what is the hook? The ego is the hook we've attached ourselves to, and we can detach just as easily.

It all comes down to one situation with two perspectives, only one of which is true. My darkest moment of looking directly at the ego's scarcity myth is reflected in a song, "Half of Nothing," I wrote. I declared:

> I *want nothing. I have nothing.*
> *And I can't give you half of nothing.*
> I *feel nothing. I am nothing.*
> *And I can't give you half of nothing.*

I wrote the song with the ego by my side, thinking it was real. I was in the depths of depression, believing that I was literally nothing, with nothing to give and no way out. Looking back on it now, I see just how accurate I was in describing the voice of the ego without my usual filters of denial. And I see how the same thought, "I am nothing," could be used by the ego to destroy me or by Spirit to save me. Thankfully, Spirit's interpretation won out in the end. Of course, I am nothing when I'm stuck with the wormy self-image I made outside of God. But cutting myself off from my Source of love is something I no longer choose to do.

FAKE IT 'TIL YOU MAKE IT

When we "give" within the world, it can easily feel false—meaning conditional or self-focused. This is perfectly logical, since it's a false world. When we resist the ego's urgings to withhold, evaluate, and give conditionally, things start to shift.

Eventually we recognize that in order to give, we must be drawing from our actual Source of abundance. There is no need to withhold what is available in an unlimited supply. There is no need to evaluate anyone's worthiness when we are equally worthy without exception. We can give unconditionally from our origin of perfection, even within a highly imperfect world, with no expectations of receiving anything in return. Once this becomes our new habit of giving, overriding the faulty one, it starts to feel more genuine as the memory of who we really are strengthens.

CHALLENGE #9

TAKE THE CHALLENGE AND BE THE CHANGE

Spirit helps us to establish trust in the abundance that flows naturally in the real but forgotten world that is our home in Spirit. We've forgotten how we set up such a terrible substitute, but remembering is worth the effort and time that it takes. The chapter concludes with this twenty-four-hour challenge: **For today and today only, I am willing to believe that I could never run out of anything that matters**.

Things I have enough of today include:

- oxygen
- money
- clean clothes
- sunflower spread
- lip balm
- Sauvignon Blanc
- friends
- sitcoms on DVR
- water
- arugula

and

- *love*

Take the plunge and try it yourself: **For today and today only, I am willing to believe that I could never run out of anything that matters**.

Things I have enough of today include . . .

LIE

#8

CHAOS IS BUSINESS AS USUAL

(so get used to it)

While the superficial truth of this lie seems hard to deny, there are some interesting hidden ego dynamics at play. "Chaos" is our unconscious acceptance that everything must change, blocking our awareness that nothing *real* could ever change. Our perfect Peace is unalterable. We often choose chaos instead out of desperation, when faced with our failure at making up a whole world that works for us. The payoff is that we get to feel like victims of countless forces beyond our control—everything from a car cutting us off in traffic, to a lover's foul mood, to a boss's need to exercise power . . . and don't forget natural disasters. Such events would be far less threatening without the element of surprise, so we've cleverly built that into the deception as well. We really should take a moment to marvel at the power of our minds to pull off such elaborate ruses.

In fact, our amnesia is the first great wonder of the world—as in: I *wonder how the hell all this happened*? The ego is happy for us to ask the question over and over again, without ever looking deeply enough to answer it. By contrast, Spirit is happy to answer it upon request.

The *Course* reminds us that Spirit can lead us into a state of *mindfulness*, wherein we constantly recognize our Source as indistinguishable from ourselves: "God is but love and therefore so am I."[1] Instead, the ego's habitual *mindlessness* denies our Source and fashions a very convincing fantasy world of chaos, driven by a fearful ethos of "kill or be killed."[2] This world can only be "real" within our wild imaginings, where we spend a lot of time struggling to make fear work better than love. (Good luck with that!)

Once there, we recognize we've made a terrible mistake and think we're going to be punished for it, so we make the chaotic world our hideout, sometimes hoping and praying that God will come and rescue us. But God is neither looking for us nor hearing our pleas, because we never actually left our Source. We're just covering our eyes with our hands right in front of the truth, while Spirit patiently waits for us to open our eyes and recognize we haven't gone anywhere.

THE ZONING-OUT FACTOR

There is a right way to zone out from life's typical stress—or to rephrase, a *helpful* way if your goal is healing instead of hiding. The wrong way is to attempt detachment by walling yourself off emotionally—even though you're still in harm's way, still believe in your victimhood, and still have no actual means of escape. The form of your attempt to escape will vary and could include raiding the chocolate stash, popping open a bottle of wine, or grabbing for the remote—anything to get an instant release from the hidden conflict within. There is a good chance this has been your choice if you feel an undercurrent of anxiety running through your life, even as you tell yourself you're successfully insulated from hurt.

The better way to zone out also involves detachment— this time put to strategic use. Here, you rise above it all completely, embracing a role as observer of the dream. Then you watch your life with Spirit by your side, trusting that all will be made clear in time, and apparent "problems" will be resolved or transformed without you jumping back into the thick of things, believing you have to apply fixes. When this trusting detachment is your choice, you feel an undercurrent of peace running through your life.

The choice is stark: you can go for utter chaos and the resultant anarchy of feelings, or you can go for the complete lack of chaos accompanied only by peace and happiness. The tricky part is that we usually make the first choice totally unawares.

LET'S ANALYZE
(lying on a couch is optional)

Learning theorist Edward Thorndike offered a simple and profound observation in his book *Animal Intelligence*, that "behavior is predictable without recourse to magical agencies." More specifically, he referred to the phenomenon that behaviors followed by desirable consequences are more likely to be repeated as the "Law of Effect."

In this respect, chaos *is* exactly what we desire. We continue to choose it because of what we get from it: it allows us to think our preoccupations are normal, while denying there is anything we can do to change our predicament (our predicament being the sum of all our preoccupations). Chaos also serves to reinforce our victimhood, solidifying our choice for self-punishment. The ego tells us that the weaker we look, the more likely we are to receive mercy instead of the executioner's blade from an angry God, when he finally tracks us down in the crazy world we created to escape him. Once again, all this is totally nuts—but you may have noticed that insanity rules the so-called world.

Another useful concept of Thorndike's is the "Law of Exercise." That means that the thoughts we use with regularity get strengthened. In this regard, our ego thoughts have developed "abs of steel," since we have overlearned them to an impressive extent. Our mistaken perception has become our reality. Chaos is a choice we make, not with joy, but with guilty desperation. Joy arrives with the realization that we no longer have to choose insanity.

THE THOUGHT MACHINE

The philosophical proposition "I think, therefore I am," put forth by René Descartes, could be more accurately stated as "I think, therefore I am a chaotic mess." Imagine a pendulum that swings back and forth between the two extremes of loving thoughts and fearful thoughts. One minute we're high with pleasure, and a few minutes later we're at the other extreme, in agony. We all know that the quickest way to stop a pendulum from swinging is to leave it alone. This would allow us to abandon the dualistic thought system of the ego altogether, gradually slowing our minds down to the still point where we accept the Spirit's thought system—which is our birthright, actually—of love and only love. But we're usually more likely to keep the pendulum swinging in order to maintain the experiences of going from one extreme to the other. Meanwhile, we may hardly notice that we're constantly going away from the still point of love, in one direction or another. That means we experience at least as much pain as pleasure, while gradually becoming more depressed as we wonder why love never seems to last.

Remembering our observer role with Spirit by our side, we can practice the *Course's* teaching of interpreting everything that happens—and everything we do or others seem to do—as either an *expression of love* or a *call for love*.

Then, even as we watch our pendulum of thought swing from one extreme to another, we can remember that the proper response to everything is simply love. We can train ourselves to see the love beyond the chaos and thus begin to live at our still center despite how crazy the world seems to be.

THERE ARE NO BENIGN THOUGHTS

It's natural to focus on our extreme thoughts of complete chaos (by not wanting them) and total peace (by wanting them to last), but all our benign thoughts in the middle require examination as well. I find these to be the trickiest of all. Right now, I can't get the new Katy Perry song *Chained to the Rhythm* out of my head. We are all "chained to the rhythm" of equating our thinking with our very survival, in the grand scheme of things. That's because what we're trying to keep alive is the image of ourselves that we've made, apart from God—where change could intrude upon the Changeless—and that requires a constant stream of thought to maintain.

This includes thinking something as simple and seemingly meditative as, "I am breathing in now. I am breathing out now." All our thinking serves the purpose of putting faith in the separation from each other and our Source. The *Course* calls for a complete and total release of separation when it suggests:

> Be still, and lay aside all thoughts of what you are
> and what God is; all concepts you have learned
> about the world; all images you hold about
> yourself. Empty your mind of everything it thinks
> is either true or false, or good or bad, of every
> thought it judges worthy, and all the ideas of
> which it is ashamed. Hold on to nothing.[3]

This is a tall order, but it is within the "nothingness," or the space between our thoughts, that the *Course* is pointing us toward that will reunite us with our True Self. Thinking does not get us there. In other words, our little self thinks, while our True Self simply knows.

KINGS AND QUEENS OF CHAOS

When we think with the ego, chaos rules the day. Spirit's correction for this faulty belief is that recognizing the oneness we never left is our salvation. As observers of the world—which is all we really are—we have the freedom to choose between chaos and harmony.

The first step is to look closely at your ego thoughts. You'll know you had one whenever you experience a loss of peace. This helps clarify the problem, which the *Course* describes this way: "You look on chaos and proclaim it is yourself."[4] Usually we choose to let chaos define us, but we can now view it as a choice that can be undone.

The second step is to truly desire something better than chaos. This happens over time, as we develop trust in Spirit's guidance over the ego. "No one who learns from experience that one choice brings peace and joy while another brings chaos and disaster needs additional convincing,"[5] according to the *Course*. We all still need additional convincing or we wouldn't be here—or *thinking* we're here. Therefore, it's crucial to spiritual advancement to be as gentle with yourself as possible. Forgive yourself for just how hard it is to consistently choose peace over chaos, on a moment-to-moment basis.

HIDE-AND-SEEK

The reason it's so hard to remember that the dream world has nothing to offer us is that the ego is masterful at convincing us that not only does it have something to offer, but also *there is nothing else.* The ego's hidden agenda is to keep us lost in the chaotic search for all the external stuff we seem to need in order to achieve completion. We don't actually know what we want, but we know that searching feels important and necessary—in part because it distracts us from the fact that we're hiding. We invest a lot of effort in finding and defending our hiding spot, lest we blow our own cover.

Looking back to the most mindless time in my life, I find the Los Angeles chapter of my story. I thought I found a moment of utter perfection when George Clooney kissed me at the Firefly Bar in Studio City, on that night I'll never forget! I can say with certainty—because I have a reliable witness in my friend Leslie—that this event did in fact happen. But even the soaring high of the Clooney kiss was short-lived, for the ego won't let you feel good about yourself for long. That's guaranteed. It wants you to never stop seeking, running, and chasing the novelty of yet another kiss. As I wrote in a song, "Perfect Rush," at the time:

> I *feel alive in the chase.*
> *You're just another nameless face.*
> I *won't be saved.* I *can't be touched,*
> *'Til* I *find the perfect rush.*

BRIDGE OVER UNCONSCIOUSLY TROUBLED WATER

You may have heard of the popular "iceberg" analogy about layers of mind. Our conscious mind can be thought of as the tip of an iceberg, above the water, while our unconscious mind, the vastly larger chunk, is below the surface and out of awareness. It is for this reason that the *Course* recommends the practice of paying close attention to the slightest irritation—because beneath it lies seething resentment, anger, and other feelings you might classify as ugly and shameful.

If minor irritations are signs of a larger problem, does that mean you are almost continuously in anger? Absolutely, yes, when you follow the ego! The thoughts and feelings you're conscious of having simply can't be trusted, for they are infused with the ego's defense mechanism of denial. It will always deny the love that you are, cherishing fear instead and proclaiming it as your identity. No wonder it's so hard to stay positive!

The *Course* equates consciousness with ego awareness, so it's not something we want to "expand." It is quite the opposite, in fact. Spirit guides us to release and let go. Ken Wapnick summed it up well in his book *Taking the Ego Lightly*:

> There is no consciousness in Heaven. Consciousness implies duality: you are conscious *of* something. There is no one in Heaven to be conscious of anyone else. There is only perfect Oneness and perfect Love and that is God. Once we believed we were separated, we became conscious.

As an aside, I'd like to give proper credit to Simon and Garfunkel for inspiring the title to this section. My parents actually got married to the song "Bridge over Troubled Water." Yes, their bridge eventually collapsed in divorce. That's not a bad thing, though; it's inevitable in the grand scheme of things. All separate alliances we make with others, at the exclusion of certain others, are on their way out—even if it is through death. This is because the idea of a separate alliance can't be sustained indefinitely, for it is contrary to the idea of perfect oneness from which we came and never left. Spirit can help us strengthen our memory of our "bridge over eternally calm water."

WHO HID MY MIND AND WHERE DO I FIND IT?

Let's start with where you will *not* find the mind you share equally with God. It is most certainly not related in any way to your body's brain, which only appears to be the source of your thinking, and unknowingly the choice for the distraction of chaos. The body's brain is simply part of the puppet body you shake around, believing it actually does things independent of the shaker/decision-maker, which is you. Our belief in it seems to bring the puppet to life, but it doesn't and never will. Which is good news, right? No worries if your puppet is not looking as good as it once did or has aches and pains, feels horrible emotions, or thinks menacing thoughts. It simply doesn't matter, once the mindless state of the puppet is understood. In other words, don't ask your puppet brain for advice—it will always tell you something crazy. Withdraw your belief in it instead, and simultaneously regain access to your real mind.

Your real mind is your home and security, a lifeline to steadfast sanity. For the sake of clarity, remember that you are an idea in the Mind of God—an extension of love without beginning or end. God did not make the puppet version of yourself; the ego did, as an attempt to extend fear and chaos as a complete replacement for love and peace, which is simply not possible.

IT'S AN EXERCISE
(mental stretching required)

This entire, chaotic, made-up world is held together by our investment in its reality. Our moment-to-moment judgments keep it all going. When we remember that we're only observers of the world and not active participants—since there is no real action taking place within an illusion—we have taken a monumental step toward restoring our sanity.

For this exercise, we will watch our mind's judgment, with the knowledge that it is only the ego doing what the ego does and will always do. Initially, our goal is not to stop judging. Judging will slow down and stop eventually on its own, once we are not invested in keeping it going.

When we're able to accomplish this "divestment" even some of the time, then Spirit has the space it needs to provide an alternative experience of knowing who we are. This alternative feels entirely different than the judging/reacting cycle. The goal is to approach stillness of mind, not the body necessarily, although bringing our bodies to rest can help minimize distractions.

Let's take an inventory of our oh-so-important upsets that mandate our immediate response. As always, me first.

SPINNING PLATES OF CHAOS

Source of Chaos	Typical Minor Imbalance	Typical Major Imbalance
The Dream World	Had to reschedule my son's birthday pool party due to rain.	Mandatory evacuation during Hurricane Sandy.
Other No-Bodies	First vocal coach let me go as a client— too many bad habits.	Suicide of a close childhood friend while in college.
My No-Body	Getting a stomach bug while on vacation in Mexico.	Making lifestyle adjustments due to asthma.
My Imaginary Feelings	Feelings of boredom on any given day (Groundhog Day Syndrome).	Feelings of depression, ranging from hopeless and functional to hopeless and dysfunctional.
My Imaginary Thoughts	"I want Gabby Bernstein's career."	"I'm a fraud, and soon you'll know."

While the sources of chaos "out there" seem to produce a range of unbalancing disturbances within me, the fact is that the seeming causes of chaos and my reactions to them are both completely external to my True Self. I can give up all attachments to chaos from seemingly external sources whenever I give up my resistance to seeing how crazy it all is and opting to watch the whole show from the still point of love within myself. Spirit chips away at our resistance upon request.

Okay, you're up!

THE WORLD IS EFFECT, AND THE CAUSE IS IN MY MIND

The examples that we came up with in each of the chart's five categories are the same, in the sense that they can all be catalysts for change. They reveal the underlying deficiency of investing in the belief that something external is happening, justifying our upsets. In my case, your case, and every case, *we are never upset for the reason we think*. The event "out there" is an effect of the cause within the mind we share: the decision to see unpredictable chaos (the ego choice) instead of consistent peace (Spirit's choice). The *Course* meets us where we are in saying:

> It is not you who are so vulnerable and open to attack that just a word, a little whisper that you do not like, a circumstance that suits you not, or an event that you did not anticipate upsets your world, and hurls it into chaos. Truth is not frail.[6]

We can't make order out of chaos at the level of the world. Order is restored when we examine our choice for victimhood and understand why we chose it—as a way to say, "Have mercy on me, God. Someone else destroyed your oneness, not me. I have irrefutable proof!" Only then can we realize that begging for mercy is completely unnecessary, since we aren't separate from God.

WE SHOOK THE SODA BOTTLE— OPEN SLOWLY

Our chaotic, mindless ego thoughts are like a shaken soda bottle. We've been shaking them since the beginning of time, with the vigor of an adolescent wanting to play a trick on an unsuspecting, thirsty friend. When we all give up this prank, that will mark the end of time. Until then, we are only asked to do our part: stop shaking our own bottle. Telling someone else to stop shaking theirs is not advised or helpful. Although I'm making an exception for myself by telling *you* to stop, of course.

When examining your own thoughts, crack the cap slowly. This will ensure a gentle experience of release vs. an explosion. It's a big leap to bring your thoughts from emotionally charged chaos to steady peace in an instant. It takes as long as it takes, and that's what time is for: to change our purpose from hiding to healing.

CHALLENGE #8

TAKE THE CHALLENGE AND BE THE CHANGE

The ego is a real BYOR party: *bring your own reality.* That's why it results in chaos as far as your puppet's eyes can see. The lesson is to remember that the *choice* for chaos came first, and now you're seeing the *effects* of that choice. Choosing against chaos and for peace has the effect of restoring Spirit's vision. With that way of seeing, you'll recognize whatever "image" before you does not define you, nor all the seemingly separate others you perceive. You, the One appearing as many, are love and nothing else. Therefore, any experience resulting in a loss of peace is a choice you made and requires your taking responsibility for it. Let's commit to another twenty-four-hour challenge: **For today and today only, I am willing to believe that I am always getting what I want, for better or worse.**

Today, my "loss of peace" moments—revealing my choice for chaos—that I'm willing to take responsibility for are:

- My daughter threw a fit while getting ready for school because of her insufficient wardrobe. She nearly missed the bus, and I thought it justified my angry reaction.

- My mom and stepdad moved into a new lake house in Minnesota this week. I won't get to see it or them for months. I thought it justified my reaction of loneliness.

What forms of chaos can you take responsibility for today? If you're like me, there's always something!

LIE
#7

THERE IS SOMEONE
OUT THERE WHO CAN
FINALLY COMPLETE YOU

(so never stop
searching)

Undoubtedly, this is another *really great lie* that's hard to give up. The search for perfect love in the form of a soul mate is at the very heart of sustaining the heartless ego. If we keep looking, it confidently tells us, we are all but guaranteed to find the feeling of completion we long for in another. After all, it's a great big world filled with endless possibilities! But according to the *Course*, the ego's secret mantra is actually "seek and do *not* find."[1] We will come up empty, frustrated, or even depressed in our search for love, because we embedded failure into the mad design of our made-up world. We just haven't looked closely at the blueprints.

What ends up happening with ego-driven relationships is really quite primitive and could be called "emotional cannibalism." The deal is: *You have what* I *lack, so* I *will devour you.* I'll let you eat me up too—for a little while. When we both eventually come up hungry for more, we'll fight about the failed promises of the menus, then find new partners and start the cycle over. Or if we're especially noble, we'll resign ourselves to an incomplete existence together, filled with starvation and chronic resentment. Either way, we get to blame our partners for failing to provide what they initially promised to deliver.

Yet all this is just a reenactment of a hidden melodrama within: *After I withdrew from the Source of Love within and created my own willfulness in place of its Will, I then blamed my Source for abandoning me.* And thus I will search endlessly for what I gave up in the first place, with whatever or whomever I find never quite providing fulfillment.

THE PRESIDENT HAS LEFT THE BUILDING

The *Course* tells us that "the symbols of hate against the symbols of love play out a conflict that does not exist."[2] I've witnessed this journey in my twelve-year marriage. When we were first living together, I was still unpacking boxes when the symbol of all my hopes and dreams lost his father to cancer. At the funeral, many were meeting me for the first time. A family friend told him, "Wow, she looks at you like you're the president!"

The ego's use of time is to keep our experiences in constant flux—even to the polar opposite of where they started. Fast forward well into our marriage with two kids, and all the pressures that come with it. I began looking at him like he was a president I didn't vote for, while hoping for the best—or the worst, depending on my degree of sanity at any given moment.

When we utilize the thought system of the fearful ego in our relationships, our thoughts are built upon a foundation of hatred. Some of them can be beautified temporarily—the *Course* refers to this as "special love"—but not permanently altered.

The way out of this is to allow Spirit to repurpose every relationship. A shift can be made from reinforcing separation wherein specialness needs surface endlessly and are never met—to accepting oneness, which releases the need for specialness altogether. It's the freedom of needing nowhere to hide and having nothing to prove.

My marriage is stronger than ever now because instead of elevating or condemning *him*, I've elevated my own awareness. This doesn't mean that specialness needs never arise or cause trouble; it does mean that they don't occupy center stage. Therefore my preoccupation is not battling over needs, but staying in my "power zone" of accepting oneness as much as my resistance will allow. Either I'm choosing the ego's hatred for myself and everyone, or I'm withdrawing my belief in it for myself and everyone. My marriage is not the only arena in which I'm doing this work, but it does give me daily opportunities to remember my choice for sanity.

LET'S ANALYZE
(lying on a couch is optional)

The work of Dr. Karen Horney, credited by many for recognizing the roots of "codependency" in the early 1940s, provides an interesting parallel to the projection of power in relationships. She described three personality types that get involved in codependency:

- "Moving toward" is characterized by compliance to a fault and involves looking for strength in dependency. Its mantra is "You know what's best for me" and takes on the appearance of sacrificial nobility.

- "Moving against" is fraught with aggressive tendencies, which look for strength via domination. In its focus on "I know what's best for you and everyone," others are viewed as past, present, or potential enemies.

- "Moving away" is displayed through aloofness, which looks for strength in isolation. The mantra of "What's best for me is my own little world" holds everyone at arm's length.

In her book *Our Inner Conflicts*, Dr. Horney expands on the notion of detachment with the clarification that when chosen consciously, "the gains to be derived from detachment are considerable." She uses the example of Eastern philosophies. But when detachment is unconsciously defended it has to do with "a fear of becoming submerged in the amorphous mass of human beings, a fear, primarily, of losing his uniqueness." This is where Dr. Horney's view converges seamlessly with the *Course*.

The truth is that we are not separate but One. There is no "other" to move toward, against, or away from. It's a push-and-pull strategy of our own elaborate construction awaiting our deconstruction, which happens merely by withdrawing our belief in it. No wrecking ball is required!

IT'S AN EXERCISE
(mental stretching required)

Since we operate as if we're separate from each other within our collective dream world, let's start where we are and take a closer look at the mechanisms at work in our own relationships. The common theme in the personality types of "moving toward, moving against, and moving away" is movement. We keep our perceptions of our relationships fluid, as a distraction from their purpose. The ego's purpose is always to reinforce our belief in separation by falsely declaring it reality. With the ego, we engage in all three types of relationship "movement," at different times in our lives or in certain roles.

Complete this chart and take a look for yourself. Try and predict what you think you'll be like at ages you haven't reached yet to get a past/present/future panoramic view.

Time Period	Overall Relationship Movement
Childhood (up to 12)	Moving Toward, Against, or Away?
Adolescence (13–19)	Moving Toward, Against, or Away?
Young Adulthood (20s & 30s)	Moving Toward, Against, or Away?
Middle Adulthood (40s & 50s)	Moving Toward, Against, or Away?
Older Adulthood (60s+)	Moving Toward, Against, or Away?

My pattern seems to have been "Moving Away" in the first two stages of childhood and adolescence. I was trying on my individuality and exploring the opportunity to define myself apart from parental influence. In young adulthood, I would say my twenties was mostly "Moving Against." I wanted to check all the boxes on my list (like marriage, graduate school, and climbing mountains—literally, not figuratively) faster and better than anyone else.

In my thirties, I was "Moving Toward," wanting to contract and hide out in my relationships for a while—unconsciously, of course. Then, a switch went off on my fortieth birthday, exactly. I shifted back to "Moving Away," but this time with a different purpose.

It was more of a soul-searching, inward expansion phase, wherein I wasn't trying to leave anyone behind, but bring everyone along as an equal. My hope is that this continues into older adulthood, because it's the only way of being in the world that feels genuine to me.

This is too much fun, right? Let's take one more look at this concept through a slightly different lens.

Current Roles	Relationship Movement Right Now
Friend	**Moving Toward, Against, or Away?**
Significant Other	**Moving Toward, Against, or Away?**
Adult Child of Your Parents	**Moving Toward, Against, or Away?**
Caretaker of (Child/Parent/Pet/Plant)	**Moving Toward, Against, or Away?**
Coworker	**Moving Toward, Against, or Away?**
Group Member (you and like-minded others)	**Moving Toward, Against, or Away?**

As I mentioned, I'm now in a "Moving Away" phase in all my relationships—as a conscious choice and not a compulsion. My intention is to "in-source" my nourishment to its actual origin, instead of source-substitutes. However, for the sake of full disclosure, I still occasionally fall into "Moving Toward" my husband, desperately wanting him to complete me (special love), and getting furious when he can't or won't. The *Course* refers to this as "special hate."[3] I would also add a third category of my own, of "special apathy." Here, I pretend it doesn't matter because I'm above it all. (Chances are that this is an ego attitude.)

I've also been known to use "Moving Against" as a group member, especially when it comes to judging those who are not spiritual seekers. My ego rant goes as follows: "I mean, what's wrong with these people? They're the walking dead and don't know it! At least I know I'm dead and am looking for life. And when I find it, they're gonna want me to tell them where it is even though they didn't do any of the work."

The ego can mask itself as "spiritual" in the blink of an imaginary eye. You've gotta love it, just for entertainment value alone!

RUNNING ON EMPTY

All our "movement" in relationships is symbolic of how we are really on the run from God. We're ducking and dodging at every pass, because we're terrified that we'll pay for usurping God's power with our own life. But we're simply out of gas on this mission. That's okay, since there is actually nowhere to go.

The *Course* encourages us to allow stillness to descend on the mind, which is its natural state, despite all the chaos we are accustomed to. Only then can we hear Spirit's call to stop moving our lifeless puppet bodies around—clinging to certain other puppets, tearing others apart, or hiding them behind our backs (out of sight, but not out of mind)—and just look at them for what they are.

We actually only have to look at one of them, and any one will do. All relationships are the same and do not change. They all, by default, serve the ego's purpose of deflecting guilt away from ourselves. Spirit tells us that this simply isn't necessary, for the separation never happened. We don't have to shake the puppets around (including the one we think is our own), pretending that they're real. They can be gently laid aside.

Laying them aside feels like sacrifice to the ego. Therefore, Spirit meets us where we are, reassuring us that we don't have to give up a thing. Spirit gladly provides a temporary service where our puppets are transformed from objects of projected hate to objects of remembered love. This is what the *Course* calls the "holy relationship"[4]—a step toward allowing love to become so strong in our lives that it no longer needs a specific object to be involved. As we realize that it is everywhere and nonspecific, we melt into the eternal love we never left.

SEX DEGREES OF SEPARATION

Where does that leave sex? Is it an act of true joining, where the two become one, or a reinforcement of separation? Well, it depends on which thought system you're using at the time. The central focus of the act is on the body, obviously, which makes it easy for us to use it to reinforce the body's reality. In *Form versus Content*, Ken Wapnick says, "Sex clearly makes the body real, whether as a way of producing children, having a good time, or as a combination of both, whether sex is guilt inducing, or a source of repeated pleasure. The body remains the central focus, and that is the real attraction."

Spirit tells us that we can't really join with another at the level of the body—no matter how advanced our puppetry skills become. It's simply not the right place to look for the completion we are seeking. We are already joined with everyone at the level of mind, the only place where it can occur.

We are not being asked to give up sex to remember our true identity, thankfully! Have it or don't have it, but see it as a symbol of choosing to join fully with another. It's no different than any other thought you have about a person, an animal, or nature when you experience the idea of oneness. It can be a thought that reflects the Truth beyond the world we made—the reality we never left.

BEYOND THE BODY BARRIER

Our little self, rooted in a body, will never achieve the experience of completion it is seeking. Our belief that our bodies provide proof of our separate existence is a belief to be questioned. Perception seems to make it so, but what can the body's eyes tell us about who we are within? They see only what we are not and could never be. The *Course* teaches that "you cannot put a barrier around yourself, because God placed none between Himself and you."[5] Our collective illusion of separation is our attempt to create and maintain such a barrier. It's a colossal mess the size of the universe, but no part of it could shatter the unity of our True Self.

I've experienced my "barrierlessness" in a sleeping dream. It was very much like an episode of I *Dream of Jeannie*, depicting the process she used to get back into her bottle. She blinked herself into the form of pink smoke, then the smoke appeared to be sucked into the bottle. In my dream, I felt my awareness expand outside the body barrier. Instantaneously, I was a part of all my surroundings. It was a feeling of complete and total relaxation, like the release of unclenching a tight fist.

Then, I suddenly felt that being everywhere was an urgent problem in need of immediate action. I thought,

Oh shit! I *need to get back into my body container before* I *wake up.* And, I felt my awareness shift from everywhere in the room back to my body, just in time. Crisis averted! God forbid I should remember that I'm actually everywhere! But God is not forbidding this recognition. Only the ego could have such an agenda, held together by our own secret desire to accept fragmentation in place of completion.

APPETITE FOR DESTRUCTION

The ego most certainly has an "appetite for destruction." Like the debut album of the famed 1980s band, the ego is always offering us "Guns N' Roses." Sometimes we only see the guns, while sometimes we only see the roses, but it's a package deal. With the ego, you have to take both. Yes, there appears to be beauty, but death is a part of it. Destruction is the mantra of choice, and our relationships reflect this as well.

This chapter's title states the lie "There is someone out there who can finally complete you, so never stop searching." The lie beneath that lie is "There is someone out there who can finally destroy you, so never stop searching." This is where the ego is really taking us, as insane as it sounds. Often, we want our relationships to be torturous because we feel we deserve to be punished. Once God catches us here, we want to be able to tell God, in a desperate plea for our life, that yes, we chose to be separate, but we didn't really enjoy it . . . it was hell! Maybe then God will show mercy. Looking deeply at the ego's hidden agenda with Spirit's reinterpretation is how we can be clear what we've unconsciously chosen for ourselves and everyone. Only then can we stop choosing it. Yes, take-backs are allowed! Every moment we are provided with another opportunity to choose differently.

We no longer have to answer the call to hate We don't have to wonder when we'll next hear the ego's call to hate, for it is incessant in the dream world. It's no match, though, for our superpower of withdrawing our belief in it. The *Course* clarifies that "love calls, but hate would have you stay. See in the call of hate, and in every fantasy that rises to delay you, but the call for help that rises ceaselessly from you to your Creator."[6]

In other words, you send out, pretend not to hear, send out again, and eventually answer your own call for help—since there is only One of us here appearing as many. If God entered the dream to answer directly, God would be making an imaginary conflict real, and would be rendered just as insane as us. The ego would love for us to see God in this way—capable of both wrath and mercy. That is how God is portrayed in many traditional religions. But this is purely a confusion of the ego, where we exchange our awareness of love and eternal life for a belief in hatred, death, and a version of love contaminated by hatred and death.

LOVE AND HATE ARE NOT AT WAR

Nothing exists outside of love. Therefore, it is not necessary for love to conquer hate. The very implication of a battle necessitates two actual opponents. Only within our collective dream could it seem possible that love is at risk—yet it is this fearful dream we secretly fight to protect.

Love is like the eye of a hurricane. The ego's chaos may swirl around us, but we can watch unaffected, without attachment. We can resist the urge to jump back into the storm, kept in motion by the guilt in our mind over the separation. Our worldly relationships may sometimes seem like a safe haven, but at best they serve only as a temporary denial of the permanent way out.

LET SPIRIT MAKE YOU A MUSIC MIX

The only real relationship we have is with Spirit, which safeguards our memory of oneness. Spirit is the "love of your life," for it contains your actual Life. Having a crush on Spirit is not required. Remembrance through restoring communication is the path. And there is a direct line of communication, if we get through our own resistance to use it.

As a music lover, especially of 1980s and 1990s pop, I occasionally ask Spirit to make me a mix tape while I'm driving in the car. I'll say to Spirit, in my head or sometimes out loud, "Okay, the next couple of songs are from you." The last time I did this on a road trip I heard "Up Where We Belong," followed by "Personal Jesus" on the radio. Very appropriate and helpful, I concluded.

I invite you to ask Spirit for your own music mix. You may not get a bliss-inducing song; I once got "Let's Get Physical." I interpreted it as Spirit making it clear that I can be taught through the physical exactly how to give up my attachment to the physical—and also poking fun at me for preferring make-believe to Reality. We laughed about it together. Spirit is always laughing! Never at us but at the idea that any of this could be true.

Spirit will gladly use anything of the world—from our favorite radio station to our favorite relationship—to help us reinterpret it all through love instead of through fear. And again, giving it to Spirit never involves giving it up. This leads us to our next topic.

LOVE AND SACRIFICE ARE STRANGERS

In the ego-driven relationship, love and sacrifice are as thick as thieves. To fill up your bottomless pit of needs, I must sacrifice my own bottomless pit of needs, and vice versa. One can easily see that there is no way this problem fixes itself. Even if your needs converge with another as a joint need, the ego will demand they diverge once again. Proof of a separate will, apart from anyone else, is part of this ill-fated bargain.

When we answer Spirit's call to remember the love beyond the ego's conflicted version of love, we begin to see an unwavering decision. There is no room for a thought of sacrifice to enter, for the idea of it has been rejected entirely. This knowledge takes us to our true power center—joining our separate will as a unified will we share with God. Here, love and sacrifice forever part. Your mantra to reinforce this truth could be "Your needs are my needs, and together we have none."

CHALLENGE #7

TAKE THE CHALLENGE AND BE THE CHANGE

Spirit reminds us that giving and receiving love are actually the same process and occur simultaneously in all instances. When I give love, I automatically receive it, because in the process of giving I prove to myself that I actually have it. Since only love is real and is endlessly available—because love is, after all, what we actually are—I constantly gain everything and lose nothing in a real relationship.

That doesn't seem to be the way of the everyday world, of course, so here comes this chapter's twenty-four-hour challenge: **For today and today only, I am willing to believe that sacrifice plays no part in love.**

My "Oops, I almost saw this as a sacrifice" moments for today were:

- Yes, I'm cleaning out the litter box . . . but that doesn't mean I'm sacrificing my own needs, talents, hopes, and dreams to do it.

- Yes, I'm eating lunch at Wendy's because the kids like it . . . but that doesn't mean I'm sacrificing my own needs, talents, hopes, and dreams to do it.

- Yes, I'm biting my tongue because my husband isn't attacking his chore list like he should . . . but that doesn't mean I'm sacrificing my own needs, talents, hopes, and dreams to do it.

Your turn!

My "Oops, I almost saw this as a sacrifice" moments for today were . . .

LIE
#6

YOU MUST FIND A WAY
TO BE TRULY UNIQUE OR
BETTER THAN OTHERS

(because you are!)

What often seems to be healthy competitiveness is, in fact, a dead end devised by the ego, whose desire for "specialness" is yet another ploy in the name of separation. If we don't continually strive to be unique and superior, the ego warns, our identity will weaken until we cease to exist as an individual at all. Spirit clarifies that only the fictional self we've created in this made-up world *would* cease to exist if we willed it so—yet therein lies the secret of happiness.

It serves us well to ask ourselves if we really want to settle for littleness here, in the world of time and space, at the expense of being aware of our glorious magnitude within the boundless home we never actually left. We can't experience both an imagined world and a true reality at once. We will go home eventually because "only truth is true"[1] and we'll eventually accept that. However, we can get there sooner if our thoughts focus on how we are the same instead of how we are different.

Unknowingly, we are constantly exercising our will to be separate from our Source. I chose to be in exile, then made up "others" for company (the kind of company that loves the same misery, that is). The apparent existence of billions of others allows one to say, "See, everyone else is separate too. It's not just me!" But it's infinitely valuable to recognize our oneness, even here.

The ego can be very tricky in distracting us from this truth. If it can't convince us to hate others who seem different—which is what it prefers—it will encourage us to join with a select group of others with common interests. While identifying with a support group can be extremely helpful in the short term, its long-term potential may be limited. If we feel that only cancer survivors, substance abusers, or parents of autistic children can truly understand us, then the ego has successfully reinforced the idea of separateness.

LET'S ANALYZE
(lying on a couch is optional)

John Bowlby's work on attachment theory in early childhood is of interest here. He believed that the ever-present threat of danger is responsible for the development of an infant's attachment to a caregiver. No one offers us protection quite like the ego (or so it tells us); therefore our own ego is really the caregiver we attach ourselves to. It seems like our best bet against the threat of annihilation, which we have feared ever since we thought we separated from our Source. The ego argues for always becoming bigger, stronger, and better than ever to keep our fear of disappearing at bay. But are we really better off with this attachment?

In Bowlby's book *Child Care and the Growth of Love*, he states that "what is believed to be essential for mental health is that an infant and young child should experience a warm, intimate, and continuous relationship with his mother (or permanent mother-substitute)." The ego can certainly claim a continuous relationship with us. It will feed us insanity as long as we will allow it. The ego is also intimate, offering a special relationship unique to you and yourself alone. It is anything but warm, though. In fact, it is as cold as death itself.

It's important to point out here that we are not born into bodies egoless. Our decision for the ego's path of separation came first within our mind. That decision resulted in the projection of our imaginary body into an imaginary world. Therefore, the mind is where the ego can be undone, if we want it to be undone. This would result in the disappearance of all bodily and worldly projections, since they would no longer be needed as proof that the impossible actually happened.

ONE-UPMANSHIP RULES THE WORLD

Before we can consider withdrawing our belief in the world, it's necessary to understand exactly how the ego rules it. The ego is always on a mission to build you up in any way possible, as a separate entity with a body borderline, to disguise the fact that you don't exist at all. It's not hard for the ego to accomplish this goal because our attachment to our special individual identities is so strong. This attachment may appear harmless, but specialness is a form of attack. The *Course* explains that "specialness not only sets apart but serves as grounds from which attack on those 'beneath' the special one is 'natural' and 'just.'"[2]

The ego's preference is that you identify with the mantra "I'm special and superior." This reflects a heavy investment in the dream world and keeps you tucked in tightly like a cocoon. The ego will gladly settle for those who prefer the opposite mantra as well, which is, "I'm special and *inferior*." Either will do, because either accepts the basic tenet that you have a separate identity and that there are "others" out there for comparison.

IT'S AN EXERCISE
(mental stretching required)

Let's examine our unconscious need to one-up or one-down on ourselves. What form has it taken for you? How invested have you become? Answer honestly with the reassurance that no one will see your list. I'll share mine, though, and will admit that I'm embarrassed at just how real I've made these comparisons . . . and how I still work to "improve" them sometimes.

MY ONE-UPS (OR ONE-DOWNS) THAT DENY MY ONENESS

I'm better/ worse than you . . .	Here's my proof!	What I'm not saying out loud.
Physically	I've been blonded by the Light since childhood. I maintain a healthy weight and rarely get sick.	Don't feel bad. I got lucky.
Socially	I often feel awkward when socializing outside my trusted inner circle. I compensate for anxiety with humor.	If you are overly friendly or boring, it's fine really. I've got a joke for you.
Emotionally	I have complete control over my emotions at all times. I never lash out in anger and am always the first to forgive.	Just don't listen to the Amazon Echo playback from when I'm behind closed doors.
Mentally	I control all my impulses with ease. As a result, I don't do anything to an excess.	It's a gift.
Spiritually	I devote time to my spiritual practice every single day without fail. I'm so frickin' peaceful. Everyone can see it!	You could try harder.

As you can see, I much prefer to be on the one-up side of things. (I threw in a one-down just to make you feel better.) Historically, I've been more invested in clawing to the top of the pyramid, claiming superiority with my list of accomplishments, than having pity parties. Whether you go up or down in your own comparisons, the reason is that bugaboo known as "low self-esteem." And that is always the ego's insane reward. Whatever our up-or-down style, we all seek recognition and constant approval of our uniqueness. This "house of separate cards" that we have placed our bets on is just that fragile and transparent. Now, it's your turn.

THE HOLLOWNESS OF VICTORY

Victory is really not that sweet, if we're honest about the experience. This is because it's isolating by nature. Our most "special" victories can't be shared. The *Course* says, "Specialness can never share, for it depends on goals that you alone can reach."[3] We don't share anything when we use the ego thought system, for we are told the opposite: that holding, preserving, and cherishing proves that you have something and deserve to hold on to it. Spirit tells us that giving freely proves that you understand the true purpose of everything.

The type of sharing that Spirit is talking about is not giving half of your french fries to your husband—which

I'm *never* willing to do. It's all about ideas, because even the physical world, your body and "self" included, is nothing more than an idea. Spirit's version of sharing is remembering our inherent oneness. We're all exactly the same, always have been, always will be. In the dream, we share the folly of forgetting our oneness, and our only need is to remember it together.

DEFENDING THE ALMIGHTY FRAGMENT

The ego will always encourage us to defend our specialness because releasing it would be death to the ego. Preserving our specialness is really saying, "Hail to the ego, death to God!" To which we reply with a resounding "Worth it!" This is only because we're afraid that as long as God lives, God will want to kill us for choosing separation over oneness. Therefore, God is the only one we're really trying to one-up. Our worldly one-ups are symbolic of that hidden conflict, which doesn't actually exist.

The *Course* clarifies: "Those who are special must defend illusions against the truth. For what is specialness but an attack upon the Will of God?"[4] Of course, God is alive and well and is the only Life we have and have never lost. We don't have to worry that we've offended God by this whole mess. We only need to let ourselves and everyone off the hook for what never happened.

BEWARE THE MARVELS OF MANIFESTATION

The ego's plan to prevent our awakening from the dream world is to keep us mindless and distracted within it. One of the most powerful ways this is accomplished is through our ability to manifest within the dream. I remember one morning a few years back when I woke up with two questions I wanted answers to. One was exactly what happened to Malala on that bus, for I'd only heard parts of her story. The other—not nearly as deep—was wondering how to make a smoky eye for a wedding I was attending. A few hours later, I was at the hair salon with time to kill under the dryer. I reached for the nearest magazine and two of the headlines on the cover were "Malala's Story of Courage" and "How to Make the Perfect Smoky Eye." I thought, *Wow, how amazing that I was able to manifest the exact answers to my questions almost instantly!*

Is it amazing though? Essentially, I made up meaningless questions and then made up meaningless answers. It just doesn't lead anywhere! It's self-contained mindlessness, just an ego trap, plain and simple. True meaning can never be drawn from nothingness.

NEXT STOP IS MISCREATION STATION

Manifesting anything in this world is like applying clear paint to a blank canvas. Our imagination fills in the picture.

In our mind, it may look like we've created a masterpiece, a train wreck, or a million scenes in between. Our work of art may fit in with others' paintings seamlessly or clash horribly. Instead of focusing on the end result—the picture we've chosen to see, which isn't really there—it would serve us to focus on the process of painting, beginning with the intention we bring to the worldly art studio.

We are creative by nature. It feels good to create, even here, and is symbolic of the only place where we can truly create—at home with God. God extends love and nothing else. God gave us the same power. Love is all we are and all we can really do. But when we're in the grip of the illusory world, we don't create; we only miscreate. Here, fear is all we are and all we can do. Yet all that's required to undo this illusory state and regain the power to create meaningfully is to withdraw our belief that it was ever possible to miscreate.

There is no need, then, for us to worry about the legacy we'll leave behind for the world when we are gone. When we go, the world goes with us. It's a package deal. This has nothing to do with the death of the body or the end of the world. Puppets and puppet stages are available in endless supply, whenever we have use for them. Our decision to give them up marks the end of the performance. Circling back to the legacy thing: love is your legacy. And you can

play that awareness on repeat in your mind . . . even now
. . . even if you just partially believe it.

I ORDERED THE SINLESS SPECIAL

The real motivation behind our compulsive demand for
specialness is wanting to project our unconscious guilt on
to others. We are certain that it's not possible for *everyone*
to be sinless. The ego's comfort zone depends upon
seeing myself as sinless but surrounded by sinners. Then
I can breathe a sigh of relief and relax for a second—but
no longer than that, for this illusory game is exhausting to
maintain.

It's like we're at a restaurant that has a limited amount
of the daily "Sinless Special." We desperately want one,
but it would be meaningless if everybody else got it too.
Either you will be saved or I will. So to hell with you! We
don't realize that this insane demand lands us both in hell.
The joke is on us because it's the very specialness of the
daily special that's poison. Only the truth, baked with pure
innocence and nothing else, tastes divine. And, of course
there is plenty of that for everyone.

BE SPECIAL OR DIE TRYING

Our True Self can never be altered, but our memory of our
eternal oneness can be obscured temporarily. Within the
dream world, we accept the falsehood that we are separate

from each other and our Source and then choose to hide this decision from our awareness. In a sense, we die to our True Self when we invest in our specialness, for they are mutually exclusive states of being.

A leap of faith is required to release our individual will, which actually has no power at all, and accept our shared will in its place. Our shared will is our saving grace. I had a dream, not long after my first time working through the Course, in which I was treading water in a rough ocean, nearly drowning, when a boat with a dozen people aboard pulled up beside me. I didn't want to be saved though. That seemed weak to me. I thought I must be out there on my own, to make a point or take a stand about something. Seeing as how I was drowning, it was hard to remember the point I was making though. The people on the boat weren't trying to forcibly pull me in. They patiently awaited my decision, looking on me with kindness and deep understanding. I realized that my choice was either to die alone—singing "I Did It My Way," like Sinatra—or allow myself to be saved by joining with my sisters and brothers. I chose joining and climbed on board.

And it's been smooth sailing ever since . . . *not!* But the dream was symbolic of a significant shift in my perception and the beginning of a gradual process of withdrawing blind acceptance of the ego. The Course reassures us by saying, "Fear not that you will be abruptly lifted up and hurled into reality. Time is kind, and if you use it on behalf of reality, it will keep gentle pace with you in your transition."[5]

THE SECURITY OF RELEASE

Surrender can be a terrifying proposition! The ego emphatically agrees and tries to convince us that our very existence will be wiped out permanently if we succumb to surrender—like we were never here at all. The ego is actually right about this, but only our dream-figure existence is at stake. And that existence will never bring us happiness.

I find it helpful to use this daily intention: "Spirit, I only want to hear your voice today. It's your voice that I trust." It is possible to quietly give up on the ego without fighting the ego. To fight it would justify its existence and actually strengthen it. One of my spiritual teachers and a close friend, John Beavin, shared this truth beautifully in his *Course*-inspired book, *The Parable of the Stars*:

> As it happened, then, it was the weakest, nearest burned-out, ready-to-give-up little stars that first learned the truth about what they really were, and they went from their sad condition to becoming the brightest and steadiest-shining stars. They didn't twinkle at all anymore, because they were not trying to outshine the others. In fact, their true brightness depended on their remembering that all the billions of stars were equal.

NONSPECIAL AWARENESS

I'm afraid we have to accept the fact that we're not really special in any way, shape, or form. We never were and never could be. We have to settle for being equal to God. That is God's will for us. Isn't that infinitely better? Not to the ego, but we are not the ego.

It may seem quite arrogant or even blasphemous to consider yourself equal to God. But, God's will for us is nothing short of perfection. It is perfection shared equally among us. If even one of us were to be excluded, perfection would slip away from our memory—as it has within the dream world.

There are three stages of nonspecial awareness. The first is to see our "sameness" within the dream world. Despite their crazy diversity, our projections are all the same in that their source is fear, and they serve the purpose of hiding. Here, we are carrying out our special mission to divide and conquer through separation, difference, and division. Spirit meets us where we are by making us aware of this unconscious decision and helps us see that it's not what we really want under any circumstances. Spirit gives us an alternative special mission: to heal through unification. Through this process, we realize that it's not really a special mission unique to any one of us; it's the exact same mission for all of us.

The second stage of nonspecial awareness is the acknowledgment that our true sameness exists outside the dream entirely in our home, which we actually never left. This knowledge results in direct access to our power center, which over time weakens our belief in our powerless center—the dream world. In this shift toward real power, our unconscious guilt over the separation starts dissolving as we develop trust in another way of perceiving. We may start with 99 percent unconscious guilt and 1 percent awareness of the love that we are; just getting to fifty-fifty would be a major feat worthy of celebration! But slowly we develop a "majority consciousness" of love, and then there's no stopping us. We will eventually be overwhelmed with awareness of the love that we are.

The third stage is . . . Well, there would be no use for words here. You are healed, whole, and enveloped in God's love, and the dream world completely fades from your awareness.

TAKE THE CHALLENGE AND BE THE CHANGE

The challenge—and, believe me, it's a challenge—is to see beyond the differences of form, to the oneness beyond it. In other words, you don't rely on perception—your senses—to inform you. You have to lower your expectations of perception to nothing, since it actually has nothing to teach you. So you stop letting your perceptions run wild, and let your higher mind rule your perceptions instead. This is done through decision making. And the only decision to make is to listen to Spirit, which is what you are.

Think of a "security blanket" of sameness. Everyone and everything fits under it without exception. The fearful ego claims that security is found in differences, specialness, and superiority, but Spirit knows that we'll only find it in the sameness of love. Love is the great equalizer, for it dissolves all differences. This remembrance is our only need.

This chapter concludes with this twenty-four-hour challenge: **For today and today only, I am willing to believe that we are all exactly the same.**

Here is my list for today:

- My yoga instructor and I share the same need.
- My brother Andy and I share the same need.

- That lobbyist and I share the same need.

- This homeless person and I share the same need.

- My dentist and I share the same need.

- This billionaire and I share the same need.

What is on your list today?

LIE #5

YOU MUST ATTACK FIRST AND OFTEN

(or risk being defeated)

cknowledging that attack certainly seems justified at times—especially after we've been attacked—it must be understood that the ego always has a hand in this primal urge. All forms of attack, from physical to verbal to just-thinking-about-it, are vehicles for the ego's agenda to reinforce the idea of separation as a fixed state of being above all else. Applying Spirit's knowledge, we can come to understand that attacking or being attacked wounds us equally. That's because there is actually only One of us here.

We are extremely resistant to seeing that truth, however, so we've invented enemies to be the recipients of our seemingly justified attacks. Not unlike the special love relationship, the agreement of enemies goes like this: *I'll try to destroy you, and you can try to destroy me. That will make each of us feel victimized and thus very important.* This weird bargaining explains why some extremely volatile relationships between opposing individuals, cultural or religious groups, and nations are maintained in vicious holding patterns that defy all logic and reason.

The ego wants us to focus intensely on our enemies. This prevents us from figuring out that it's actually our unconscious guilt over separating from Source (that never really happened), which is behind attack in every form. As the *Course* reminds us, "You are trying to escape a bitter war from which you have escaped. The war is gone."[1] We won't experience this truth, however, until we take a closer look at the guilt within.

ALL ROADS LEAD TO GUILT

Our thoughts are like the roads we travel on our time and space trip. It is extremely telling to simply watch your thoughts and see how quickly they circle back to guilt. The guilt may be displaced on to others (*How could a terrorist blow up a building with people inside?*) or placed squarely on ourselves (*How could I say such a terrible thing to my own child?*). We may even have guilty thoughts that appear relatively benign, like *Why did I buy Colgate toothpaste when I prefer Crest?* Subtle guilt is just as much of an indicator, though, of what looms under the surface of our conscious thoughts—the guilt we are not yet willing to look at because of our intense fear.

Guilty thoughts have a highly addictive quality. Speaking for myself, I rarely go more than five minutes without one. I've tried to suppress them, but that gives me the feeling of holding my breath underwater. I'm fine at first and then panic sets in, forcing me to admit that I need guilt as much as I need air to breathe! We all do. It's a package deal when we believe our identity is anchored in our separate bodies. And most of us have made an unconscious decision that the payoff of an individual existence is worth the guilt.

I even catch myself planning guilty thoughts I'd like to have in the future. It's smart, really, like a savings account. We need guilt on reserve for a rainy day, don't we? For instance, when I was thinking about my approaching birthday—my personal Declaration of Separation day—I decided that I wouldn't remind my sister Lisa, one of my closest friends, about it. If she forgot, and I was hoping she would, then I'd have a reason to feel guilt at her expense. And I *actually breathed a sigh of relief at the thought of it.* This is what we do, as childish and manipulative as it sounds. She did, in fact, forget my birthday, but it didn't feel as good as I had hoped! Deep down, even deeper than where we choose guilt, we actually don't want it at all.

GUILT MAKES THE WORLD GO 'ROUND

We've all heard the saying *"Love makes the world go 'round."* The ego thought system replaces that with *"Guilt makes the world go 'round."* The *Course* says, "Love and guilt cannot coexist, and to accept one is to deny the other."[2] We have a choice to make then. We either come from a place of love, seeing the innocence in everyone that lies just beyond what we perceive with our senses, or we don't. This is easier said than accepted, for sure.

The *Course* teaches us that we are guiltless in Spirit. There is a part of us that knows this to be true, but then there's the problem that we're still here in the land of guilt—guilt as far as the eye can see. It's similar to the anthem that goes "This land is your land; this land is my land." In this case it's "this guilt is your guilt; this guilt is my guilt. This guilt was made for you and me." Sharing is all we can do. We can only share what is true, though—which includes innocence; but never guilt, except in a dream.

THE BROOM OF DOOM

Since guilt feels so terrible, we are desperate to get rid of it. We'd like to have a broom that could magically sweep it out in any direction away from ourselves. This would provide immediate, although temporary, relief from our dire situation. We may admit a little guilt ourselves but remain secretly delighted by the comforting idea that others are guilty of worse things than we are. Regardless, any degree of guilt means we are essentially at war with the world and ourselves. If taken to the extremes, it can explain the unconscious thought process behind a homicide: "All guilt is yours, and you must be destroyed." It also can shed light on the mentality of a suicide: "All guilt is mine, and I must be destroyed." The *Course* cautions us that it's dangerous to think that death can bring peace. Only undoing our self-made fear at its source, the ego, can do that.

The goal is to make a conscious choice to refrain from sweeping altogether. Sweeping is psychic busywork, being preoccupied with pushing away a problem so that we don't actually take the time to understand it. Wait . . . does this give me a spiritual excuse to stop cleaning my house? (Ha! It's worth a try.) While there's nothing to be gained from closely examining the dirt in my house, there is something to be gained by closely watching our guilt, instead of trying to sweep it away whenever we notice it. If we can see the patterns of its formation, then we can devise a strategy for undoing it and gain a permanent restoration of our spotless innocence.

Obviously, we have a complex relationship with guilt. We are constantly attempting to resolve the inner tension of not wanting the guilt—because it doesn't feel good—but also realizing, at an unconscious level, that if all the guilt was gone our individual identity would go along with it. This prospect is utterly terrifying! Our choice, then, really comes down to innocence in oneness or guilt in separation—although the latter is only an idea we thought was worth exploring and then decided it wasn't. We aborted the mission long ago, yet have the ability to pretend it's an option now.

LET'S ANALYZE
(lying on a couch is optional)

An interesting parallel can be drawn from the work of Dr. Thomas Harris and his popular self-help book from the 1960s, I'm OK—You're OK. There he writes about morality and concludes, "The Golden Rule is not an adequate guide, not because the ideal is wrong, but because most people do not have enough data about what they want for themselves, or why they want it."

In transactional analysis, a therapeutic method, the core belief is that our social interactions reflect our understanding or misunderstanding of ourselves. Typically we occupy one of four states of being, namely:

1. I'm OK—You're OK
2. I'm Not OK—You're Not OK
3. I'm OK, You're Not OK
4. I'm Not OK, You're OK

Of these, I'm OK—You're OK is the only desirable state, which can also be interpreted as I'm Not Guilty, You're Not Guilty. With Spirit guidance, you alone can restore oneness when you see yourself as innocent and reach the same verdict for all others without exception.

The other three states of being all involve our tendency to project guilt outward on to others, or inward toward ourselves. Gary Renard, an international *Course* teacher, has made the observation that Westerners often display a pattern of an outward projection of guilt, while Eastern cultures are more likely to project guilt inward. Either form is detrimental, and either form can be corrected once understood.

It's possible to achieve a state of false peace when all guilt is projected outward or seen as outside of yourself. This would be I'm Not Guilty, You're Guilty. Then you are essentially at war with the world and you see yourself as an innocent victim. You feel powerless, but you're unaware that you are using your power to keep yourself in this state. It's a complete refusal to look inward, and isolation is the result. It's an acceptance of your little self (ego identity) and complete denial of another option. Children, who come into the world ego intact—by their own choice—operate this way. My son recently blamed me when he stubbed his toe because I called him into the room.

Most of us mature relatively quickly into the next state: I'm Guilty, You're Guilty. We are willing to accept guilt on some occasions, but pass the buck as well. At war with ourselves *and* the world, guilt seems very real here. We see it in ourselves and in everyone. There is an element of joining with each other but not for the right purpose. Because of the "joining" piece, it almost seems an acceptable practice or status quo. This stage will continue until the following idea enters our mind: "Is it possible not to feel guilty or make others guilty?"

We all reach the next state eventually. It involves recognizing the war is within. Here, all guilt is projected inward where something can finally be done with it. It's called I'm Guilty, You're Not Guilty. This is a very delicate state in which you really don't want to hang out alone. Spirit can carefully guide you through it. You are correct in identifying yourself as the source of your suffering, but Spirit will tell you that nothing has really happened. You just thought you were something it wasn't possible to be . . . guilty. Your complete and total innocence has never been in jeopardy. The action necessary is to simply change your mind about the idea of guilt.

From the mind-set of innocence, we come full circle and return to the state we've never left: I'm Not Guilty, You're Not Guilty—although the "I/You" distinction disappears completely with the remembrance of oneness as our True Self and permanent state. I've presented these four stages as if they were moved through in one lifetime or one dream. It's more likely that it takes many dream lifetimes—one after another—to get there. There is no difference, though, between a singular or serial dreamer in the ultimate sense, since time itself is part of the fantasy. And fantasy has no power over Reality—not even for a moment. Amen to that!

IT'S AN EXERCISE
(mental stretching required)

Together, let's reflect on these four states of being and how they operate in our own lives. You may be wondering, *If we're actively looking for guilt, won't we find more of it simply because we're focusing on it?* In fact, we've already chosen to put guilt absolutely everywhere. That part is already done. Now we need to choose to remove it from absolutely everywhere. Ripping a colossal Band-aid off all at once is quicker than uncovering each individual wound.

We have to start somewhere though. For most of us, our default setting is to pretend that guilt resides within certain others to varying degrees, while others—ourselves included—are somehow spared. This "selection process" covers up our secret demand for guilt under all circumstances. Complete the chart below to reveal your guilty pleasures that always result in pain, the pain of losing sight of your innocent True nature.

State of Being	Circumstances Most Likely to Produce It
1. You're Guilty, I'm Not Guilty	
2. You're Guilty, I'm Guilty	
3. You're Not Guilty, I'm Guilty	
4. You're Not Guilty, I'm Not Guilty	

1. I'm most likely to project guilt outward when I think of the political scene, nationally and internationally. I'd also have to include big corporations and Big Pharma in this category as well. The bigger they are, the better they are for me. Then I can say, "Well, what could I possibly do to stop them? I'm just one person." The dividing line of guilt and innocence remains clear.

2. I like to share guilt with someone I share a goal with, like my coparent/husband. Our mantra is "We will most likely screw up the kids, but at least we'll do it together."

3. I take on guilt myself when I think of my career aspirations, which have been, until now, in the fields of psychology and music. I've clung to the belief "It's my glory if I succeed and my guilt if I don't. Either way, no one can take it from me."

4. Only with a spiritual focus have I approached seeing the innocence in myself and everyone. This is a new anchor for the rest of my judgments as well, leading them all toward nonjudgment.

Similar to a "No-Fault Insurance Policy," we can adopt a blanket "No-Fault Innocence Policy." The ego will resist this declaration because guilt is pleasurable to the ego. That's why we ask, "What's your guilty pleasure?" The idea of guilt is the pleasure, and any form of it will do. The ego will tell you that you never have to give up the guilt and shouldn't trust anyone who suggests it. The ego is aware that it began as nothing more than the idea of separation and had no power until we attached guilt to it. The ego weakens as we begin to withdraw our guilt.

Spirit can help us detach from the guilt altogether, which is not the same as denying it. To deny it would be to make it real and then cover it up. Spirit restores our awareness that our innocence was never something we could throw away. It's an inalterable, eternal, God-given state of being.

LETTING THE WORLD OFF THE HOOK

The world is never going to do its part to bring us the freedom of peace because we set it up to imprison our peace. Think of it as a court of law. The world according to the ego is like a prosecutor charged with establishing irrefutable proof of guilt directed at horrific victimizers at the expense of helpless victims. And we will continue to witness guilt-inducing events—even referring to some of them as acts of God—as long as we think we're here. Specific examples could be provided, but focusing on specifics is part of the problem—preventing us from seeing the big picture. Guilt is not outside (in the world) and out of my control, but rather inside (my mind) and completely under my control.

Injustice is in the mind of the dreamer of the world. The world can only follow the strict orders we've given it. The ego keeps us unaware that we first condemned ourselves to hell over our decision to separate from our Source. Then, to ease this unbearable burden, we created the world in order to escape our personal hell for a collective hell, because that would enable us to claim permanent victim status. The *Course* tells us, "What you behold as sickness and as pain, as weakness and as suffering and loss, is but temptation to perceive yourself defenseless and in hell."[3]

I know that Billy Joel felt otherwise when he wrote his song, but we *did* start the fire that's been burning since the world's been turning. The fire—our unconscious guilt—came first, and the projection of the tumultuous world followed.

PEACE FLOWS LIKE A DISTANT MEMORY

We decide how much peace we are willing to accept—in other words, how much we are worthy of receiving—on a moment-to-moment basis. It may start with a trickle as we hesitantly test the waters, but we can allow it to expand into a broad river of remembrance. Spirit tells us that peace is our natural state and that barriers to peace are of our own construction. It's simply not necessary to maintain an elaborate defense system against the peace that we are, since no other alternative exists.

Fear—our constant state of being with the ego—can make this remembrance a seemingly impossible task. The *Course* provides clarity with the declaration "How foolish to be so afraid of nothing! Nothing at all! Your defenses will not work, but you are not in danger."[4] It follows then that we can either be vulnerable in fear or invulnerable in peace. In practice, when I experience a loss-of-peace moment, I say to myself, "I must not feel completely worthy of peace right now, but I can choose again. Peace flows through me with ease. It can be no other way without my consent."

BREAKING THE GUILT BARRIER

Once upon a time, we had a shared goal of breaking the sound barrier. Breaking the guilt barrier would be a far more useful goal to pursue now. It's the unconscious part of the guilt that's tricky. How can we remove what we're not aware of? How can we remove what we have an investment in keeping hidden? We can't do it alone, but yet it must be done. Spirit can help us remove guilt without feeling shame.

Think of it as an intervention orchestrated by the Highest authority. The truth is that our eternal innocence is guaranteed by God. It doesn't always feel that way, does it? Have you ever had a feeling of doom and gloom for no apparent reason? That's unconscious guilt. Again, we put it there, not God, and we can remove it with help from Spirit, which is our own memory of oneness with God. It's important to realize the power you have in this process. You are not a helpless victim, although that is a role we often play in the dream for the purpose of deflecting guilt.

Looking at our guilt in action is the path toward transcending it through understanding. This is possible through our unconscious use of projection. Because I suppress my guilt internally—meaning I don't claim it as my own—it appears externally as yours, in the form of something you did or failed to do. If it seemingly originated from you, than I can conveniently "forget" that I used you as a storage space for my own guilt. Of course, this only works when I accept the ego's insistence that you and I are separate. Spirit's gentle reminder of our oneness leads me to another conclusion.

HASHING IT OUT OVER HASH BROWNS

Breakfast is my favorite meal of the day, and perfect hash browns are one of my reasons for living. I'm talking dark-brown hash browns smashed onto a griddle with a weighted press and coming out like a giant potato snowflake. Well, only one restaurant in town knows how to make them. It's a spendy place overlooking the river, so I don't go often.

But I wanted to go one morning when I had a long to-do list and had just been told by my husband—lovingly, of course—to watch our budget. Of course my ego answered that advice with "No one tells me what to do." I ordered the hash browns, but there was definitely a side order of guilt in my mind. When the hash browns came, all I could do was laugh. I was served hash *grays*, not browns—pale and pasty cubes of potato, not crispy strings. And they were loaded with steamed peppers and onions, making the presentation as soggy as it was smelly.

I knew in that moment my guilt had ruined the whole thing. It had nothing to do with me not *deserving* the perfect hash browns, and it wasn't the fault of the waiter, chef, or food supplier. I had already condemned myself to "hash grays" before I sat down. The world simply responded to my unconscious request for self-punishment. My Spirit-guided awareness of what was really going on prevented me from being upset for more than a few moments. The goal, then, is to be willing to look at upsets as an opportunity to heal. If I had viewed myself as a victim of the "hash gray" conspiracy, I would have blocked that opportunity.

I AM THE ASSASSIN I AM HIDING FROM

Having kept a dream journal on and off for thirty-five years, I've experienced endless displays of victimhood as a common theme within my dreams. Sometimes it's subtle; I once dreamed that I was taking a college class but wasn't given the room number, so I was forced to wander around the building in confusion. Other times it has not been so subtle, like when I dreamed I was being pursued by a gunman and was hiding under a table, with my heart pounding out of my chest, trying not to make a sound.

This will certainly sound insane, but when I recently had my first dream where I was the assassin, I viewed it as quite an advance! Symbolically, it was a personal breakthrough for me to see myself as the victimizer with the power—to destroy with the ego or choose again with Spirit—instead of the powerless victim not capable of anything but suffering. Since there is only One of us here appearing as many, there is only one metaphorical gun, and in my dream I could have put it down for everyone. I didn't, of course, I was too frightened! I could have, though, and hope to sooner rather than later.

It's important to remember that the undoing of fear itself is an active process and that we are working with ideas as agents of change. We are urged by Spirit not to passively accept the ego's way of thinking, where avoiding attack thoughts directed at ourselves or others would be an impossible mission. We are meant to question our ego alliance, which is the same as saying we are meant to question our acceptance of our little self. When we do, we can ask, "Why do I think it's possible to attack?" That question changes everything as we slowly realize that it's not!

COLLECTIVE DISARMAMENT

Each of us has the power to end the war for all of us, since we're essentially playing all parts simultaneously. It seems as though we're only a fragment of the whole with a fragment of the power. But our part contains the whole, since separation is not possible. Mentally, we can retrace our steps back to where we first believed it was possible to take steps on our own in order to run, hide, and defend ourselves. From that place, we can choose the opposite instead: to stand still and not defend ourselves. Here, we join together armed only with the memory of our oneness and fully recognize our shared goal of peace.

The ego insists that defenselessness is weakness and the worst possible choice, but the ego's version of anything is never the whole story—and always nothing more than a story. Spirit assures us defenselessness is where our true strength lies and is the only choice in reality.

We can stage a peaceful campaign that starts with our own thoughts (for action automatically aligns with our thinking). It's a realization that the attack/counterattack cycle will never end until someone decides to stop, and not out of superiority, but rather a recognition of inherent equality in oneness. To take this idea all the way Home is to understand that when I attack, I attack no one but myself. I no longer want to pretend that's possible, since thinking I can seems to rob me of my birthright: permanent peace.

CHALLENGE #5

TAKE THE CHALLENGE AND BE THE CHANGE

It's necessary to put forth willingness—and even a slight willingness will suffice—to relax our defensive impulses. These defensive impulses stem from the belief that we've been attacked by others, are currently being attacked, and will be attacked again. You can see that this faulty belief conveniently covers the past, present, and future, so there appears to be no escape from the necessity to defend ourselves. Far beneath that layer of erroneous thinking is the belief that we attacked our Creator in order to experience a separate identity as our own creator. This explains the guilt surrounding all our creations in our illusory kingdom, for we think we've stolen every single one. And we fear retaliation is inevitable and justified because that's how we respond to threat. Our Creator does not share in the fear behind attack, for it is not real.

This deep level of understanding is necessary before we can become open to the prospect of truly healing our illusions. The *Course* makes the declaration "Here is the gift of healing, for the truth needs no defense, and therefore no attack is possible."[5] We have, in fact, maintained our complete and total innocence throughout our entire dream state journey. We just overlook it often and fall back into the pattern of assigning guilt.

In practice, it's easier to see innocence in certain people over others. Collectively, we project innocence on to babies and the elderly once they return to a babylike state. It's the years in between when we damn each other and ourselves to hell, like that was a normal and possible goal to achieve. Spirit leads us toward a new shared goal of seeing innocence in everyone. No one can be excluded since we're not really separate, even now.

Open yourself up to the slightest possibility that your innocence is something you can count on. It just might be true. You'll know you're seeing yourself as innocent whenever you are able to see the innocence in others.

The twenty-four-hour challenge for this chapter: **For today and today only, I am willing to believe we are all completely innocent.**

Here is my list for today:

- I see complete and total innocence in this school bus driver. (Difficult: When my daughter was injured on the bus, I didn't feel he handled it well.)
- I see complete and total innocence in my cat, Zane Grey. (Very easy: My cat can do no wrong in my kingdom!)
- I see complete and total innocence in this store clerk. (Easy: She was pleasant and helpful.)
- I see complete and total innocence in my girlfriend Kelly. (Easy: We have so much in common, it's ridiculous.)

You're up—what is your list for today?

LIE #4

THE PERSON WHO CAN HOLD A GRUDGE THE LONGEST WINS

(so hang on tight!)

The ego will cheer us on until we hold *the last grudge standing*—the ultimate prize. It's a mantra of "Only the weak let things go!" If we do, against all odds, attempt to release a grudge under the ego's guidance, it will be of little value. Whether we do so because we're better than anyone who wronged us, or we demand an apology with a dramatic ultimatum, or we hide a lasting resentment behind momentary kindness, in each case we have still fulfilled the ego's goal of seeing ourselves as separate and better. Even when we muster up enough compassion to understand where the other character in our grudge story might be coming from (although that's an improvement), what would really cut to the quick is to acknowledge that a part of us—the false part—unknowingly consented to the story with the goal of self-punishment. And, wow, was it ever effective!

Spirit can help us unlearn this style of destructive forgiving with a reminder of oneness, which means that all forgiveness is self-forgiveness. As the *Course* teaches,

"My grievances show me what is not there."[1] Any grievance against another is symbolic of our totally unjustified grievance against our Source: *that it somehow wronged us when we forgot about it.* Can we laugh about this yet?

OUR GODSIZE GRUDGE

We most certainly *do* hold a grudge against God, consciously or not, whenever we think with the ego. I observed this with my daughter Aubrey. She was seven years old and in trouble for something I can't remember, when this conversation ensued:

Aubrey: "I'm SO mad!"

Me: "I can see that. Are you mad at me for taking away your stuffed animal?"

Aubrey: "No, that's not why I'm mad."

Me: "Are you mad at yourself for playing a part in this?"

Aubrey: "No, I'm mad at God and I don't know why. I don't want to be."

I was shocked and powerfully moved by her response. It was so raw, honest, and unsolicited. We had never talked about being angry at God—quite the opposite, in fact. So I had no choice but to punish her further for such an atrocity against her Creator! (I'm kidding, of course.) Her revelation instantly opened up a dialogue between us. I told her that I think we might all be secretly mad at God, but we can be open to the idea that we're wrong about what God has done or failed to do. If God can only love and we were created from love, then that's probably all we're able to do.

IT'S AN EXERCISE
(mental stretching required)

Let's take a look at our grievances, big and small—and believe me when I say I'm dreading this as much as you are. Who wants to see their petty yet always seemingly justified grievances in one place at the same time? That is precisely how to deal with them though: to gather them up in one basket, so we can see what has led us to become basket cases.

It feels like each of our grievances is locked in a separate vault in the past. And they would be dead, buried, and gone if we would leave them be. But we give them new life each time we bring them into the present by thinking about them. We believe they require safekeeping, for the ego is very invested in keeping them safe for posterity. The more grievances—in number and severity—that we invest in, the more the ego thrives. The ego's business is to eventually have you accept that you are a lost cause and beyond repair. The ego knows it's more likely to convince you someone else deserves that judgment. The ego is fine with that too! It's really a removal of hope in your mind that it's after.

Let's start by looking at our upsets with the world. It's easier to look at grievances we hold at a distance as the world's problems than to look closer to home at our own. An exhaustive list is not necessary. Instead, aim for a representative list, from a minor irritation to complete and utter horror. The benefit to looking at the deepest, darkest grievances is that we can use our *outrage* to come *out* of our *rage* permanently. I'll go first.

I wish this never happened *to the world.*	Reaction Rating Scale: (1 to 10) 1=sparking, 5=flaming, 10=raging
The Holocaust	10
The Great Pacific Garbage Patch	7
Acid-wash jeans	1
SPAM (in all forms—cyber and meat)	4
I wish this never happened *to me.*	Reaction Rating Scale: (1 to 10) 1=sparking, 5=flaming, 10=raging
Rejection by the man I identified as my one and only soul mate in 1999.	8
Rejection of myself during the dark days of postpartum depression in 2009.	9
Rejection by Captain Kangaroo, who never sent me the free coloring book I ordered in 1977.	2
Rejection by the only Powerball ticket I ever bought in 2015.	1

Now it's your turn. Use additional sheets of paper as required. I'm not judging (much).

Your list most likely includes a variety of hurts across the reaction rating scale, like mine. The first step to transforming them is to look at them all without judgment. With this awareness, we can begin to see them as all the same. Grievances of all degrees are exactly the same in that they represent a self-inflicted barrier to remembering the truth of who we are—love and nothing else.

In processing my list further, as soon as I included the Holocaust, I honestly felt a twinge of disappointment. I knew I'd never be able to top that one with my own personal list. When we think with the ego, there most certainly is a competition over who has endured the most suffering. It's considered a badge of honor. But the truth is that it's helpful to see the commonality in the confusion. We're all suffering all the time when we believe in the world's reality and nothing else. Spirit gently reminds us that it's a dream life, with no connection whatsoever to our actual life.

With forgiveness, we can transform our dream of despair to hope and even happiness. The *Course* says, "The dreams forgiveness lets the mind perceive do not induce another form of sleep, so that the dreamer dreams another dream. His happy dreams are heralds of the dawn of truth upon the mind."[2] The truth is fully recognized by our choice for love over dreams of hate. Our other option is to trade certain grievances for certain others with an unwillingness to let them all go, which keeps the illusion *alive*—as if that were really possible.

LET'S ANALYZE
(lying on a couch is optional)

Few psychological theories have included perspectives on forgiveness, for it was long thought to be too closely tied to religious beliefs. The lines of spirituality and psychology are certainly blurring more now than ever, but the seeds for what is now called "transpersonal psychology" were planted some time ago. Carl Jung, Sigmund Freud's contemporary and wayward student, was superior to his mentor perhaps only in his willingness to look beyond the little self to acknowledge the True Self. Jung believed that forgiveness was inextricably linked to one's perspective on the situation. He drew the analogy of viewing a situation from the top of a mountain to actively gain clarity.

But this higher perspective may seem paradoxical at first. In Jung's book *Modern Man in Search of a Soul*, he states: "The unexpected result of this spiritual change is that an uglier face is put upon the world. It becomes so ugly that no one can love it any longer—we cannot even love ourselves—and in the end there is nothing in the outer world to draw us away from the reality of the life within." To clarify, this higher perspective doesn't cause the world to appear ugly, but rather reveals that our ugly ego thoughts produced ugly effects—and from the higher perspective of our choice to think with Spirit, instead, becomes all the more accessible. Spirit thoughts are eternally linked to our Source of Love, which is not of this world.

ABOVE THE BATTLEGROUND

The *Course* provides a similar analogy, of viewing the world from *above the battleground*, where our purpose shifts from seeking to conquer to seeking to understand: "The senselessness of conquest is quite apparent from the quiet sphere above the battleground."[3] The ego conquers either by triumphing over other people, or, when this can't be done, surrendering to them—with a corresponding grievance etched in stone.

Spirit reminds us that giving up the battle entirely is the only way out. Using the metaphysical awareness that no one has wronged you—because no one else is here—is helpful. Realizing that you have not even wronged yourself—because you are not here either—is even more helpful. It is necessary to fully acknowledge how much we cherish our public and private battles before we can give them up. This is no easy task and requires us to forgive ourselves for how completely unwilling we are to do it most of the time.

Merely entertaining the idea that forgiveness might work better is the starting point. Releasing the belief that letting go of grudges is hard is helpful, because holding on to them is much harder. You have to remember to stay in character no matter what. And there is only One of us here playing all parts simultaneously. That means you are angry victim#6, angry victim #5,801, and angry victim #2,999,999—just to name a few. Would you give it all up if you knew you could? I can say that I'm committed to trying. The thought I'm reaching for is "What do I get out of thinking it's possible to be a victim?" In other words, what purpose does it serve?

THE LIGHT BEYOND OUR GRIEVANCES

It takes conviction and more than just a little willingness to explore the depths of our unforgiving thoughts. My grievances literally change me into something I'm not and never could be. Ask Spirit to join you, to ensure you've chosen love as your interpreter instead of fear.

The ego leads us to believe that it provides the service of hiding our darkness—from ourselves, others, and God—when it actually hides our light! The payoff waiting for us at the end of this journey is unimaginable. Even though it's a gusty morning, I'm looking at the trees and they are clapping for me. The entire dream world unites to support this goal I will inevitably choose. This happens when I flip the ego script "The world and everyone in it is out to get me" to "The world and everyone in it is here to cheer me on."

All forgiveness is ultimately self-forgiveness. Each time you forgive a seeming "other," you are calling a truce with yourself. When you're unable to see the light or innocence in another, it never has anything to do with them. It's a message from you to you, that you are unwilling to see the light in yourself in that moment. With the next moment, though, comes another opportunity to get it right. We can't fail at this, for our Light is not extinguishable. It came from outside the dream world entirely—the home we never left.

THE MIRACLE FORGIVENESS OFFERS

I remember one of my first misperceptions about how the world works. I was a preschooler at the time and thought that wind was caused by the trees flapping. Thankfully, I was corrected before sharing my theory with too many people. I was right about the cooccurrence of tree flapping and windy conditions, but I reversed the cause and effect.

Reversing cause and effect is precisely the error in perception that the ego makes constantly and Spirit attempts to point out to us. Our decision for separation and the denial of oneness is the cause and the world (the projection resulting from that decision) is effect. The world could never be causal, even though it always appears to be. In other words, we are *always* upset because of the choice for separation that we don't remember making. We are *never* actually upset about anything happening in the world at large or the part of the world we carve out and call our own. This is where forgiving ourselves for getting it wrong comes into play. And usually it takes a miracle for us to admit that we're wrong!

THE REJECTION OR PROTECTION OF FORGIVENESS

The ego rejects the idea of forgiveness entirely but will play along with our attempts with the confidence that they'll most likely end in failure. As long as our will to be separate is in play, we will fail. Simply thinking there is an "other" out there to forgive is enough to keep the ego's script going. We know we've chosen this path of *unforgiveness* when we experience an array of negative emotions along with it.

In Ken Wapnick's book *The Arch of Forgiveness*, he states, "Whenever anything disrupts our peace, we know we have left the arch, and then all hell breaks loose. However, we need only come back and peace will return, for within the pillars of safety, we know that nothing outside them can affect us." Forgiveness offers us the protection we are seeking. It is not weakness, but a return to the strength of unity. Either we're all forgiven or none of us are. It doesn't work any other way.

I'll use my dad as an example of someone who I used to kick out of my kingdom with ease. This banishment has included attempts on my part to keep him from my doorstep and my mind. After practicing the type of forgiveness that the *Course* is talking about—that is so complete and total—I honestly can't even make myself upset with him anymore, even if I try. And I have really tried to, just for the sake of experimentation. A memory will come to mind that used to be a trigger, but the visceral reaction just doesn't follow. And it feels amazing!

THE GRIEF WITHIN GRIEVANCES

It certainly seems like our grievances deliver undeserved grief to us. They are often so complicated, with unexpected twists and turns, requiring obsessional levels of vigilance just to figure out exactly who deserves blame and how much. It is never any individual grievance that is the issue though—or the whole lot of them, for that matter. Each grievance is symbolic of our grief over the separation from our Creator that we believe actually happened. This represents an unconscious denial of what we are: inseparable by design.

Within the dream world, we are most definitely grieving the love we think we threw away. Little do we know that outside the dream, we remain united in the love we could never lose.

The awareness of the purity and constancy of this love is beyond our comprehension—because the images of our dream world were created to deny and oppose it. Our experience of the images we see, though, can and will shift from fear-inducing to love-remembering. Each grievance we are presented with is another opportunity to make this "paradigm shift."

Holding grievances is like stretching a rubber band. Even the smallest investment in ego thoughts of separation automatically adds tension. In the case of a grievance that makes your blood boil, it's the equivalent of pulling the rubber band to its limit, with the likely result that it will snap back at you.

We may not be ready to put down the rubber band for good, but we can train ourselves to hold it loosely. Resist the urge to add additional tension by stretching it, even though you want to *snap* someone good! Ask yourself, Do I *really want to snap myself over this*? That is essentially what you're doing in every case.

Punishment in all forms—withholding love, eye rolling, the cold shoulder, the middle finger, Twitter rants, etc.—are simply things we pretend to do to distract us from what we know we must do eventually . . . forgive it all. The *Course* says, "Forgiveness is the only sane response."[4] (There are no qualifying statements after that declaration.) It is for One, for all, and for always.

FORGIVE LIKE IT NEVER HAPPENED

Speaking of elasticity, it's time to put on your stretch pants and feast on the true nourishment of forgiveness with total disregard for who "deserves" it—because everyone does. Forgiveness is the only dish served in the spiritual buffet line, for it serves a higher purpose. According to the *Course*, "Forgiveness is for God and toward God but not of Him."[5] God has no use for such a concept, but we do, until we feel worthy of accepting our place as equal to God.

Our forgiveness must eventually reach a level so total and complete that it is like a blank slate. Nothing from the past is carried forward. Nothing from the present is anticipated. Only the present choice for forgiveness is held on to, briefly, until even that is no longer necessary. I use this affirmation before going to sleep at night:

> I *forgive the world for what never happened.*
> I *forgive myself for desperately wanting to make it all seem real.*

It's possible that I use this affirmation at night because it frees me up to hate people as necessary during the day. Hey, it's a work in progress for all of us! I do know that when I'm making a grievance *real*, I'm *real* sure you're the one in need of correction! But I want to focus on my own correction work exclusively, for I know it's the only way out of the cycle.

JUDGE TO YOUR EGO'S CONTENT

But what if you just can't do it? Forgive, that is. What if there are a handful of people whose crimes just can't be expunged from your record? First of all, great job with the honesty thing! Thinking you've forgiven everyone and everything is most likely a form of ego denial. The ego prefers you never forgive, but if you're on a forgiveness mission, it will hasten to announce, "Great job! You're done!" That way you will quit prematurely.

Second of all, go ahead and hate if you must. The problem isn't really hating people; it's *thinking that hating is an option*. Who is "out there" to hate? It's just the One appearing as many—all versions of you. No need to hate yourself either though. Because you're not your ego—never were, never could be.

Thus your hateful ego thoughts are not to be feared. They have absolutely no power at all. They are nothing. They can't save (certainly!), but they also can't condemn. Just leave them be, peacefully. The whole thing will dissolve on its own—quicker, in fact, if you're not beating yourself up in the process over not being able to let them go.

The difficulty level is set by your imagination. Think that it's extremely hard, and you're right. Think that it could be less hard, and you're right. Think that it's easy . . . and most likely the ego is chiming in again. E*asier* is a realistic goal. Spirit can work with that.

THE FORGIVENESS CLASSROOM IS NOW IN SESSION

We can repurpose the world from the ego's torture chamber to Spirit's forgiveness classroom, wherein we are ready and willing to examine our faulty perceptions about everything. Instead of active fault-finding, our interest shifts to recovering faultlessness. This mission hinges on choosing the right teacher—Spirit over ego.

The ego teaches through punishment and lacks the insight to evolve. Spirit allows us to be happy learners in the worldly classroom. This occurs over time as the ego's fear tactics are unlearned. We must look at each one, though, leaving none of them hidden away "in case of emergency." Our willingness to look without judgment, alongside the right teacher, is all that's required.

YOUR PERSONAL JUDGMENT DAY

It's not a difficult task to witness the ego doing what it does. The difficult part is realizing that the dream world is in fact *all ego, all the time*. Soap operas don't disguise this at all and actually present the ego on speed! No one gets to be happy for long—often only from one commercial break to the next. I happen to be a third-generation *Days of Our Lives* watcher—for research purposes only, of course! It's ironic that they are called *soap operas* when all they do is air out dirty laundry—no soap is ever actually involved. Grievances are fast, furious, and rarely resolved.

One of my original songs, "Judgment Day," was played on *All My Children*. I wrote the lyrics before committing to a spiritual path of looking inward, and the song is reflective of a time when entertaining fantasies of revenge was sweeter than chocolate! I can see why the show's producers thought it would fit right in. Here is a sample:

> *You left me so anesthetized*
> *by all of your compulsive lies.*
> *I feel so justified.*
>
> *Someone needs to teach you a lesson,*
> *read your rights, hear your last confession.*
> *Can't let go, wanna make you pay.*
> *Your time has come, it's judgment day.*

If we indulge this kind of revenge fantasy, it's always directed outward at some criminal mastermind. Your personal judgment day occurs when you realize that you alone, clinging to your desperate separation from God, are the mastermind involved. But Spirit assures that you could never be a criminal. In the process of reuniting with thoughts of God, we can finally lay to rest the idea that we, the innately Godlike, could ever depart from eternal, all-encompassing love to seek the paltry rewards of revenge.

CHALLENGE #4

TAKE THE CHALLENGE AND BE THE CHANGE

The reason that forgiveness can be so incredibly difficult is that we unknowingly cherish our hurts. Each individual hurt is symbolic of the fact that we cherish *hurting* in general. The ego wants us to believe we deserve it and can't escape it. Just looking at this misperception without judgment can take the sting out of our hurts now and actually protect us from experiencing future hurts as well. The *Course* reminds us that "Forgiveness paints a picture of a world where suffering is over, loss becomes impossible and anger makes no sense."[6]

The twenty-four-hour challenge for this chapter: **For today and today only, I am willing to believe that I can let go of anything that was done to me or that I have done**.

My forgiveness lessons for the day are:

- I ran out of hot water this morning while showering. Grievance filed against the contractor who owned our home prior to us and flipped it with cheap appliances.

- I thought about my mom today but didn't take the time to call her. Grievance filed against myself for not making family a priority.

- I made an effort to cook an above-average meal tonight for the family, and no one seemed to notice my extra effort. Grievance filed against my ungrateful husband and children.

- I only got a few comments on today's Facebook post, and I felt it was worthy of more. Grievance filed against my Facebook friends for failing to document the approval that I so desperately need.

What are your forgiveness lessons for the day?

LIE
#3

REACTING OUT OF FEAR COMES NATURALLY

(so stick with
the program)

Operating in fear is our default setting until we choose to follow Spirit—the Teacher of love—instead. "Fear and love cannot coexist,"[1] as the *Course* puts it. We are either loving or fearful all the time; only the ego believes it's possible and necessary to mix love with a healthy dose of fear for our own protection. But love built on a foundation of fear is doomed to fail. Fear mixed with love is our experience only because we set it up that way—the cruelest form of self-punishment imaginable. And we *are* just imagining it—a continuous reenactment of believing we discarded love and must fight fearfully to get it back.

When we operate from our little self, it's our own power that we fear the most. This is because we feel we misused it already, resulting in catastrophic devastation of the state of perfect oneness. This irrational guilt is the motivation behind our seeking refuge here in the world, and it's why we continue to pretend we're powerless to many forces beyond our control from moment to moment. The ego tells us that our power is not always accessible and produces unreliable results at best. But when we are tuned in to our True Self, it becomes crystal clear that blindly following the teacher of fear is not the best course of action unless the paralysis of fear is our goal.

FOR FEAR'S A JOLLY GOOD FELLOW

To the ego, there is no greater companion and trusted friend than fear. It is always there when called upon. And it is always called upon, for there is nowhere else the ego can turn for reinforcement. Even the ego's version of love is built on fear. From within this perspective, there is no escaping fear. But, thankfully, we can watch our fear and we have the power to reject it.

Spirit has no animosity toward fear and its seeming effects, simply not recognizing it at all. The *Course* instructs, "Fear is a judgment never justified. Its presence has no meaning but to show you wrote a fearful script, and are afraid accordingly."[2] It's an important step to recognize just how frightened we are at *all* times, when we think with the ego. Our childhood fears of the past have not really left us; we just attach them to current circumstances. It's less realistic to try working through them all than it is to release the very idea of fear.

In practice, when you catch yourself in the midst of any negative emotion, you can say to yourself, "Oh, I'm listening to the wrong teacher. This is the fear script again." Then allow your emotional reaction to pass. It will pass surprisingly fast if you don't invest in it further with your attention. Think of it as having no more significance than a YouTube ad that pops up and says you can Skip Ad in 4 . . . 3 . . . 2 . . . 1. Watch it count down, and then hit Skip on the ego's advertisement for something fearful without getting sucked into experiencing the whole thing. A more peaceful . . . centered . . . calming . . . loving thought is *always* behind it, because that state is permanent. It's only our own interference that enters in— at our own invitation, although it rarely seems that way— preventing our awareness of love's presence.

LET'S ANALYZE
(lying on a couch is optional)

Joseph Wolpe is best known for his work in treating phobia, an anxiety disorder where someone will go to great lengths to avoid a feared object (like a spider) or situation (like flying in a plane). His method is called "systematic desensitization" therapy. The intent is to diminish an overly sensitive fear response to an acceptable level. First, the client makes a rank-order list of the least to most feared ways of coming into contact with this object or situation. Then, the client learns relaxation techniques and uses them to work through their list.

In the case of a snake phobia—of which I may have a mild form—I might be asked to imagine I'm in the opposite corner of a room with a snake in a glass case. Then, I would visualize walking slowly toward the snake, touching the glass, and maybe even the snake. All of this imagery is done while using deep relaxation techniques, focusing on the physical body.

The point is that this process works in part because it is slow, gentle, and gradual. That's what we need, as well, and what Spirit can provide—a trusted Voice of reason to help us undo fear at its very source. Otherwise, it's likely that we'll replace the feared "snake" with some other symbol of fear in the dream world.

Let's apply this method of desensitizing our fear of our own power in a systematic way. Initially, I can acknowledge that when I see a situation as out of my control, my fear is seemingly kept to a minimum. This is because I feel no one can blame me for a wrong decision if I wasn't allowed a decision at all. Spirit's coping technique is to tell me that it's safe to take it further.

The next level, even though it reveals a considerable amount of fear, is to understand that I can always control my reaction in any situation where I experience a loss of peace. And that is no small feat! Spirit's coping technique is to suggest that I refrain from attack thoughts toward another even when they appear to be justified, while forgiving myself for how difficult it is to do so.

To take it even deeper, I can realize, even though it reveals a tremendous amount of fear, that not only do I control my reaction, I control the entire situation itself. I am playing all parts of it at once. And that is one colossal revelation! Spirit's coping technique is to suggest, again, that I refrain from attack thoughts—this time directed at myself—while acknowledging how difficult it is to do so. Spirit can even reveal why I would want to play this game and attempt to fool myself in the first place. I'm told that the fear I experience is merely the outer reflection of my own inner desire for self-punishment over the destruction of perfect oneness—which never actually occurred. In my mind, I substituted real life with the board game called "The Game of Life." And I'm definitely getting bored with it!

In Wolpe's book *The Practice of Behavior Therapy*, he shares a difficulty he experienced in working with some clients who could not visualize beyond a certain point and instead appeared to "detach themselves from the imagined situations, viewing them as if from the standpoint of a disinterested spectator." He saw this as a negative outcome, a lapse in focus. I would argue that this is the goal for all of us: to detach from imagined situations (and all of them are imagined) and view them as if from the standpoint of a disinterested spectator. That's perfect! Again, we have to be quick to forgive ourselves, though, for how difficult it is to detach from fear that we would prefer to see as reality.

SHADOW CHILDREN

It can be helpful, although often unpleasant, to visit the frightened child within. It's important to realize that our inner fearful state is anything but accidental. It is most certainly willful on our part. We only pretend not to know the source of our multitude of fears—which is really just one fear: that we will be annihilated for our choice to separate from perfect oneness.

The *Course* is prepared, metaphorically, to hold our hand through the shadows of the past to help us experience a present, fearless calm: "When a child is helped to translate his 'ghost' into a curtain, his 'monster' into a shadow, and his 'dragon' into a dream he is no longer afraid, and laughs happily at his own fear."[3]

As counterintuitive as it may seem, the fact is that our darkest fears simply do not exist, and our experience of them dissolves upon contact with the light of Spirit, our memory of the oneness we never left. Our willingness to recognize when we are fearful is the first step. Looking at our fears without judgment is the second step. Eventually, we'll see every seemingly different form of our fear as having the same content.

For example, my fear of losing my husband and being alone is similar to an "inner child" fear of being abandoned by my parents. This can be traced back even further to an "inner child of God" fear of being abandoned by my Creator. On the family tree of fear, all of the branches are connected to this original fear based on the incorrect assumption that separation—and therefore abandonment—is possible.

Over time, these connections will be more apparent to all of us, as our willingness to look at what we've kept hidden expands. Until then, it can be helpful to look at our fears separately—especially any that have blown up to epic proportions and taken on a life of their own. It's important to remember, as we go through this together, that our fears are not alive and well. They represent nothing more than misunderstandings that most certainly can be corrected.

IT'S AN EXERCISE
(mental stretching required)

Let's head straight in the direction of our fears. They are rooted in the past, but linked to the future in the sense that we are afraid our past transgressions will spill into our future by being repeated. And they most certainly will when we allow the ego to have its way with our thoughts. If we uncover the constancy of the ego's tactics, however, we can crack the code.

The purpose of this exercise is to get in touch with the pervasiveness of our fear. It is ever present and strangles our awareness of the present moment. This robs us of the capacity to see anything as it is now, instead mistaking it for something that once was, and that we fear will be repeated. It takes a mighty willingness to look without judgment at this consistent hidden pattern of behavior we all share. We think we can at least be sure that we want our future to be better than the past. But the ego's "fear gone wild" thought system can produce a panicky response regardless of outcomes, for that is its goal! Fill in the chart below and take a look. I'll go first.

And now you're up, my fearless companion! Remember that the goal is not to manufacture an imagined fearful response where there is none. The goal is to realize that fear is always there, though we can certainly choose to deny it. Seeing it clearly and choosing not to believe in it is the way to release it—from a specific situation at first, until we learn to generalize the lesson and apply it to all situations at once. We are either totally fearful or totally incapable of fear. There is no middle ground.

When I was completing the chart, it was not at all difficult to think of the "accompanying fearful thought" related to a positive or negative outcome of an event that I deemed important. Fear gets us either way! The important lesson is not to stop there out of desperation. Upon request, Spirit

FUTURE FEARS INVENTORY

Life Category	FUTURE EVENT: with a negative outcome	Accompanying Fearful Thought	FUTURE EVENT: with a positive outcome	Accompanying Fearful Thought
Relationships	My marriage ends in divorce.	"What if I'm all alone?"	My marriage stands the test of time.	"What if I'm resigned and unhappy?"
Work	My first book is a failure at launch.	"What if I could have done more?"	My first book is a success.	"What if I can't keep it going?"
Leisure	I never get to travel the world.	"What if I stay trapped at home?"	I get to travel the world.	"What if I get robbed or contract a disease?"
Fate of the World	Institutional corruption goes on unchecked for centuries.	"How many people will suffer?	Institutional corruption is rapidly exposed across many sectors.	"What if we all lose faith in humanity?"

can help us find the healing aspect embedded in any feared outcome.

Our Teacher of love reminds us to consider the *purpose* behind everything. The ego's purpose is to *make alone through fear*—which is easily accomplished, since fear is not real and therefore can't be shared. It's naturally isolating in that way. Spirit's purpose is to *unify by undoing the fear* and that's all. In the absence of fear, love as our permanent state of being is remembered. When we feel ourselves in the grips of fear, making it very *real*, we can simply reach for the ego's kryptonite—that is, Spirit's awareness of the changeless Truth that the very idea of fear is impossible. Your inner "super-Spirit-hero" knows the way—time to Spandex up!

EACH FEAR IS RELATED TO EVERY OTHER FEAR

The *Course* says, "Produced by fear, the ego reproduces fear."[4] This reminds me of the computer science concept of GIGO (Garbage In, Garbage Out), which simply states that faulty input yields faulty output. Our faulty input was accepting the fear-inducing idea that separation from each other and our Source was possible and was what we wanted above all else. All output following that decision has been infected with fear and is therefore faulty.

We shouldn't be the least bit surprised when we observe the ego doing what it does, what it has always done, and what it will always do. We can learn from its predictability and consistency. It serves us well to remember that the ego is not only an unmotivated learner but completely incapable of learning. When we keep our expectations of the ego appropriately low, we'll see it for the manipulator that it is. When we raise our expectations of the ego, thinking it deserves to be given just one more chance, we're on our way to being fooled. Fear cannot be transformed into love, but we can change our mind about the decision that gave birth to it.

The most productive route is to pay attention to how you and others you observe use fear to divide and conquer. Also, notice that fear beckons us to fix our attention outward. The ego, our teacher of fear, wants to keep us focused on worldly problems and worldly solutions. Looking for possible solutions in an impossible world simply doesn't work. We can use such situations to lead us inward where the solution lies in the form of changing our own perception.

I'll share the inner dialogue from an entry in my *Catalog of Fears: Spring 2017 Edition*: "I'm really afraid my aunt's cancer will return. I wish there was something I could do. I read something about an alkaline diet making a difference. It sounds hard to follow. I don't think she could do it. I don't think I could do it. My stomach hurts. I can't imagine going to her funeral. How many funerals have I been to? I'll never forget the first one when . . ." Then I recognize that my thoughts are spiraling out of control with fear. I must be sharing this experience with the wrong teacher.

I ask Spirit for help in seeing this differently, so I can spiral back into control. The Voice of insight allows me to see that I fearfully perceive my aunt as separate, fragile, and in need of change because that is how I fearfully perceive everything and everyone, including myself. Could I instead take comfort in the possibility that we are indestructible and eternal, even though the opposite seems to be true? In this moment I think I can, but I can't speak for the next. This is not easy stuff!

I do know that it's worth the effort to secure my own Spirit connection first, before trying to be of service to anyone else. It's similar to securing your own oxygen mask on a plane before helping others. Whenever we come from a place of completion—a feeling that things around us may change, but there is nothing that must change—we automatically extend that comfort to others. Healing effects will be received by those involved, and those not even involved, because of the connection we share.

A DREAM OF RECOILING IN FEAR

A few years back I had a dream that made it clear to me just how deeply I can resist healing. In the dream I was curled up in the fetal position, feeling completely abandoned and without hope of being rescued. I reached out my hand anyway, just in case someone I wasn't able to see was there to help—someone from the "other side." I was immediately flooded with anxiety that someone might actually grab my hand to help me! I instantly jerked it back to my comfort zone of isolation.

The ego was designed to hide out of fear. Healing is unknown to the ego and therefore feared. Thankfully, we don't need to wait for a search-and-rescue party to arrive. Healing begins at our slightest invitation. We don't have to "do" anything to reacquaint ourselves with the love we never lost. "Doing" is of the ego. Spirit's focus is on "being," and we only have one option. Since only love is real, love is automatically experienced when we don't try to be anything else. We're always reaching for the goal of fully remembering the truth of who we are, a truth that can only be denied temporarily.

FORGIVING OUR ATTACHMENT TO FEAR

Forgiveness is part of the healing process every step of the way—not just in relation to releasing grievances—although it starts that way. We eventually need to forgive our attachment to fear itself. We've become so tolerant of fear that we accept it without question. This is perfectly acceptable to the ego, but we're learning not to trust the teacher of fear to lead us away from fear.

Let's check in with ourselves and ask, "What's my fear baseline?" Overall, how fearful are you when your eyes first open in the morning on a regular day? And by regular day I mean one where you're juggling a few minor-to-moderate-level crises but nothing of a catastrophic level. On a scale from "1 to the character in *The Scream* painting," what's your fear baseline? I would say mine is currently 3. I think it's been as high as 9. Obviously, the benefit of a lower baseline number is that you have more wiggle room to handle the aftermath of a major fear bomb. The good news is that even moving one point down the scale yields noticeable effects. It takes motivation to stay on top of it, though, so it doesn't creep back up. And this is where we have to forgive ourselves for how hard that can be.

FEAR HAS A SHELF LIFE

The truth is that the only part of us that has a shelf life is our fear. It's on the way out, and the ego knows it. In fact, we've already completely awakened from this dream where everything dies. Forgiving ourselves for ever believing fear could take the place of love was the final eye-opener. We're able to pretend, though, that we're still in the dream fighting for our lives. This is a decision to see only the past—and the impossible past at that.

My literary mentor and established *Course* teacher D. Patrick Miller shared the following insight in *The Forgiveness Book*: "Forgiveness blossoms at a certain moment in time, when you are ripe and ready to release some of the dead past. It is the intent to forgive that actually speeds up time, collapsing old schedules of suffering and bringing unimagined possibilities inestimably nearer." In other words, it doesn't have to take an eternity to remember we are eternal.

This concept of collapsing time reminds me of my favorite Prince song, *Raspberry Beret*, where he sings, "She walked in through the out door." The second we entered the dream world was the second we exited the dream world. We actually never really entered it at all; we merely entertained the idea of it, ever so briefly.

NO FEAR FROM HERE

When we follow the ego, we make an unconscious decision to fixate on our past regrets and future anxieties exclusively, such that the present moment is completely inaccessible. The ego knows that if we had any sense of "now," we could use it to choose against fear at its source. For this reason, Spirit gently directs us away from past regrets and future anxieties toward the present moment, our decision-making power center. Once securely in the present, we can stop actively choosing against love.

In a sense, each present moment is an opportunity for "birthless/deathless" awareness that we appear to be in the world, but we are not of it. I realize this is an abstract concept, and it may be difficult to feel grounded in it at first. It gets easier as you allow Spirit to show you that your connection is not to anything specifically in varying degrees but to everything to the same degree. For example, I may feel most connected to someone who looks, acts, and thinks like me. Spirit reminds me that I'm just as connected to someone who appears to be the opposite of me in every way. In this light, no one is required to change to be seen as the same.

Peacefully observing the dream world, without believing our role is to judge it, is the goal. In practice, it's similar to the experience of Magic Eye 3-D art, wildly popular in the 1990s, where you looked at a seemingly random jumble of colored dots but were rewarded for holding your gaze patiently at the center of the image with the intention of seeing through it. Only then would a hidden 3-D image eventually appear. The hidden image is the experience of oneness—not seen with the body's eyes but felt at a core level. And it can only be felt when a decision is made to look past all seeming differences.

FOUR STEPS TO FEARLESS FREEDOM

From the vantage point of Spirit awareness, there is no fear. It's hard to imagine living that reality, but I'm told it's possible. I'm starting to actually believe it's true. What I do know for certain is that eradicating fear is an inside job. The world doesn't do its part to reduce fear, but it doesn't produce it either. Fear is produced in the mind by our decision for it and is reflected in the world.

The other choice is to remember that love flows naturally in the mind when we stop producing fear, and this love can be reflected in the world as well. This doesn't magically make the world real but provides feedback that our fear-production efforts (even the unconscious ones) are winding down. At some point they will cease entirely. Until then, we can caffeinate the process with these steps:

FOUR STEPS TO FEARLESS FREEDOM

F   **Forgive** yourself for losing your peace.

E   **Exit** the ego, your investment in fear.

A   **Accept** Spirit, your remembrance of love as your identity.

R   **Realize** love was your only option all along . . . and enjoy!

The goal is to reduce the time it takes us to see the love beyond our fear. Seeing the fear is a necessary part because we put it there, and therefore we need to remove it. In this process, it becomes obvious that we've bound ourselves to fear by letting ego be in charge. Spirit tells us we've allowed fear to become our *new normal*, and we only need return to our *original normal* of love and nothing else.

CHALLENGE #3

TAKE THE CHALLENGE AND BE THE CHANGE

This chapter's twenty-four-hour challenge: **For today and today only, I am willing to believe that my power is unlimited and extends beyond what I can see.**

- I see love beyond this frustrated child's demands.

- I see love beyond this desperate advertiser's rant.

- I see love beyond this stress-inducing mortgage statement.

- I see love beyond this playful squirrel outside my window.

- I see love beyond this calming sunset.

For today and today only, how can you believe your power is unlimited and extends beyond what you can see?

LIE
#2

LOVE IS A SIGN OF
WEAKNESS AND CAN
REALLY MESS WITH
YOUR HEAD

(avoid it at all costs!)

The ego's goal is to use fear to block love in all forms from our awareness and then send us on a desperate, never-ending search for it. The ego doesn't want us to remember that we are love itself. If we did, the ego would cease to exist instantaneously. The *Course* encourages the mantra "Love is my heritage, and with it joy."[1] We can learn to tell which MO (modus operandi) we are following by how we are feeling. Our feelings, though, are not typically straightforward—almost never, I would contend—and need to be sorted out. We can feel either with Spirit's constant clarity or with the ego's shifty, self-defeating murkiness.

DRUNK ON THE FEAR/LOVE COCKTAIL

The ego likes to keep us constantly impaired with an elixir of fear and love. Sometimes it tastes sweet and loving, while other times it is bitter and hateful. Either way, ingesting it damages our ability to think clearly. Or, more accurately, it impairs our ability to *choose* clearly. The ego tells us that fearful love is the best type of love we can hope for, while Spirit reveals that constant and all-encompassing love can have no opposite.

Denying our fear is not an effective option. What we keep hidden *does* affect us greatly. Collectively, which really means the One of us here appearing as many, we've made the decision to look. Sometimes this can be experienced as things getting worse before they get better. That certainly seems to be true when looking at current events in the world. Fear in all forms is being uncovered at an accelerated pace, reflecting our decision to no longer allow it to hide. We can only heal what we identify as in need of healing. Spirit can help us understand that hate speech and hate crimes reflect self-hatred of an unimaginable intensity. The only self we can hate, though, is the false one we made. We share the ego that keeps that lie going, and we share in the responsibility to look beyond the lie to the Truth, where the only thing we experience with an unimaginable intensity is our happiness!

FOCUSING ON OUR COMEBACK RATE

Popular *Course* teacher and love enthusiast Gabrielle Bernstein talks about the concept of a "comeback rate" in her book *The Universe Has Your Back*. She says, "Our happiness is a direct reflection of how quickly we can restore fear back to love." That can be a measure of our progress on the spiritual path of remembering our True Self as love and nothing else. The kind of upset that previously took days, months, or even years to bring to a peaceful resolution can eventually require only minutes to transform. Because love is the inevitable landing site, this process is natural and hastens when we get out of our own way.

The "comeback rate" is a process of identifying your own personal patterns of moving away from love into an unnatural state of fear. For me, this plays out in my "I'm not a good parent" script. I'm aware now that I assigned this script to myself before even leaving the hospital with my first child. (I've never been one to procrastinate! LOL!) If anyone even suggested in passing that there might be a better way to feed or discipline my child, I would replay it in my head for years—no exaggeration. Those were my two biggest triggers because of my son's feeding issues since birth and behavior problems since preschool, both of which I blamed myself for causing and maintaining. I allowed this story to build and gain power. I collected evidence from this witness and that witness to support my failure to change the situation. The only way I started to change it, though, was to look at it differently. I made the connection that I was choosing to allow fear to take me to its happy place—suffering. And that I could choose to stop! I have thoughts and feelings of being a bad parent far less frequently now, and when I do, it just doesn't stick. I use self-talk like, "My worth is in no way determined by me. It is established by One who knows that I am love and nothing else. And in this I trust."

LET'S ANALYZE
(lying on a couch is optional)

Carl Rogers developed a therapeutic technique known as "unconditional positive regard." It involves showing complete support and acceptance of a person no matter what that person says or does. This is comparable to what the *Course* is asking us to do. We are meant to practice seeing past how someone appears to be, which can shift from moment to moment, to the changeless perfection beyond it. It's a perfection we share equally with God, for that is God's will. Granted, it's an easy task to think of Mother Teresa as equal to God, so start there. Just know that to exclude anyone is to exclude everyone, because of that oneness thing that we just can't get around even in our dream of being separate.

I'm getting an image of the famous Oprah episode where all audience members were gifted with a new car. She exuded joy when she pointed and shouted, "You get a car, and you get a car, and you get a car!" Seeing only the perfection in someone is the greatest gift you can give anyone. It means you're willing to really see them. While this mind-set can maximize our spiritual growth, it's difficult to maintain when we have only experienced *"conditional positive regard"* for ourselves.

Within the world we made (the ego's domain), experiencing conditional positive regard is really the best we can hope for. It's likely that we'll also experience the true colors of the ego, which is "unconditional *negative* regard." No one here is entirely excluded from outpourings of hate, and there is no one we hate more than ourselves. The ego offers escape from this pernicious thinking by creating a hostile world to take the blame. We have forgotten, though, that we are only imagining a state of being where we are separate from our Source of Love. And imagining doesn't make it true. Spirit can guide us back to our repressed memory of perfect and total innocence, where no one is excluded from outpourings of love.

In *Client-Centered Therapy*, Rogers describes a precursor to psychological maladjustment where "there takes place a type of distorted symbolization of experience." The maladjustment we share began with our choice to put more faith in fear than in love. When we look at the world, each other, and ourselves through the lens of fear, we can't help but distort what we see into symbols of hate. Our distortion is so all-encompassing that we literally see nothing as it is. Spirit can help us practice looking at everything through the lens of love instead, without distortion. It's possible to experience the perfection we share even within the imperfection of the dream world. We need this step to reestablish our trust in love. Our part is simple. We're only asked to no longer want to keep our unloving thoughts. If we can honestly say we don't want them, that's enough.

FOLLOWING THE STRAIGHT LINE

On my father's childhood farm in rural Minnesota, my grandfather would put blinders on his work horses, Dick and Babe, to help them focus their attention in one direction: forward. Spirit can provide this function for us upon request. Trust is required, and Spirit will earn it quickly by showing us how much easier it is to release fear and experience the love beyond it when we go right through the fear instead of around it.

This doesn't mean we turn a blind eye to the world and do nothing but selfishly focus on the thought that this is not our home. But focusing on the truth that no one can suffer, die, or be excluded from the love that we share equally with God can make us more effective in the world. This is true because we've healed our perception of it (giving up fear for love) and changed our purpose from hiding to healing. We need only to allow our trust in Spirit to outweigh our trust in the ego. In a song I wrote called "Straight Line," I explored this very conflict:

> *Draw me in. Give me a reason.*
> *Your promises need follow-through.*

Pulled me in every direction.
Need a straight line to You.

Although I wrote this song as a desperate plea to connect with another person, I am certain as I can be that my real plea was to reconnect with Spirit. I capitalized *You* to reflect this awareness. I'm happy and willing to be shown what love is by One who knows, for it's abundantly clear that I have tried and failed on my own.

OUR LOVE HANDICAP

Similar to a golf handicap—or so I'm told, since I don't play—we all share a love handicap when we think with the ego, which again is our belief that we could be separate from each other and our Source. It's a handicap that doesn't vary. We are all equally incapable of understanding love within the ego's thought system of separation. This is completely by choice—a choice to experience love's opposite through the complete and total denial of love. The *Course* clarifies:

> *You do not know the meaning of love and that is your handicap. Do not attempt to teach yourself what you do not understand, and do not try to set up curriculum goals where yours have clearly failed. Your learning goal has been **not** to learn, and this cannot lead to successful learning.*[2]

In this regard, the ego's efforts are utterly commendable *and* condemnable! We can first acknowledge the cleverness of this scheme, which is of our own design. (I'll pause here so we can pat our own backs.) Then we can opt out of the ego's loveless song and dance that promises perfect love, while secretly assuring that no real connections will ever be made under any circumstances.

A helpful affirmation might be "Spirit, I have been love-poor for far too long. Help me to remember and experience my natural state of being love-rich once again." I'm rolling my eyes as I write this, not just because it's corny but because I suspect that I don't really want it—not 100 percent anyway. In other words, the impoverished love that I know is less frightening than the abundant reign of love that I don't know.

LOVE HAS NO SUBSTITUTE

Our Source does not recognize partial love in any form. Our Source would never conceive of withholding love from anyone or anything. Our Source could never imagine making demands of sacrifice—or allegiance for that matter—in order to prove one's faithfulness to love. We are the ones who are playing around with those ideas.

Like our separate will, which doesn't really exist, we can get in the way of the sun's rays. But the sun is unaffected.

The sun doesn't cease to exist if we can't sense its presence. Likewise with love.

The *Course* instructs, "Love offers everything forever. Hold back but one belief, one offering, and love is gone, because you asked a substitute to take its place."[3] It's important for us to ask ourselves under what circumstances we are allowing ourselves to justify love's substitute—hate, which is best understood as fear. We can learn from the dark shadows of our own making that we can't help but be in the path of light and love. There is no other choice. Therefore, our judgments about others, ranging from the most loving to the most hateful, are meaningless and futile.

IT'S AN EXERCISE
(mental stretching required)

Let's examine this idea further by applying it to our own inner circle of family, friends, and beyond. By this time, we know that Spirit would have us check every box in the chart on page 174, under the column "Unconditional Positive Regard," while the ego would prefer we check every box under "Unconditional Negative Regard." Let's give our egos the chance to fill out the chart, since it's so eager to make judgments. Right? The goal is not to silence the voice of the ego but to listen to what it's *really* saying, so we can wholeheartedly choose against it.

LET'S PLAY "REGARDING YOUR RELATIONSHIPS"

Unconditional Negative Regard	Conditional Regard (+ or -)	Unconditional Positive Regard
	husband	son & daughter
	parents	siblings
	friends (childhood/ college/work)	
	public figures (world/ religious/business/ entertainment leaders)	
	complete strangers who cross my path	
me		
		my pets (living & deceased)

The pattern I see with myself is that I project "innocence" or "unconditional love" on animals and children—my own and my siblings, whom I also think of as my children, since I was much older when they came into the picture. Before having my own, I used to think I loved all children. Now, I know that's not true. I think I've exalted my own, and I only like your kid if he or she is nice to my kid. With most "others," I checked the "conditional" box, with the attitude of "Show me that you're decent, and I'll be decent in return. I'm not going to be decent first though. I'm not crazy! What if I open myself up for manipulation or abuse?"

The ego assures me that is smart thinking! And now it's your turn.

So what do we do with this observation of the ego in action? Well, we can transform it—and we have to, because no one can do it for us. I've always had the gift, or curse, of being able to trace any wrongdoing or negative outcome in the world to myself, acknowledging my small or large part. I rarely let myself off the hook for anything I experience. That has felt very punishing over the years, but I think that mind-set of responsibility has also helped me on the spiritual path. We *are* on the hook for imagining things the way they appear to be. Thinking someone else has that power can give us a break, of sorts, but it will always be unproductive. Resisting the urge to displace or project responsibility brings faster, long-lasting results, including peace of mind.

LOVE AS THE GREAT EQUALIZER

It's time to dig deep and *really* affirm the work we've just done. The *Course* declares, "Love is one. It has no separate parts and no degrees; no kinds nor levels, no divergences and no distinctions. It is like itself, unchanged throughout."[4] The hierarchy that each of us builds in our mind—specifying whom we're going to love, from least to most, minute to minute—simply isn't going to get us anywhere. Either we decide to love everyone with Spirit or we decide to love no one with ego. We can define the ego as *a completely loveless state of being*.

Spirit's alternative is a completely love-filled state of being. Loving everyone in totality means seeing through whatever fearful, offensive costume they might be wearing at any given moment, and seeing the unalterable purity beyond it. It means understanding that *purity* is what bonds us, and that it is a bond that can't be broken.

Think of it like handing out Halloween candy. We give it freely and equally to all of the children who come to our door, even though we prefer some costumes over others. Some costumes are adorable and some engender fear. Fear is just a very popular, overused costume that we can choose to wear or choose to shed. We certainly don't need to ask someone else to take theirs off to prove they are love underneath. We *know* that on some level and can act accordingly.

Since there is only One of us here, appearing as many, imagine that you are the only person holding the candy bucket *and* the only kid getting the goodies. You can give out candy unconditionally to all the other versions of yourself. In doing so, you alone would transform fear to love on a grander scale than you could ever imagine! And, yes, I'm saying that candy equals love. Have you tried Skittles?

ENERGIZING OUR EXPERIENCE OF LOVE

During my yoga teacher training, I experienced my heart center in a way that brought me closer to understanding my eternal nature as love and nothing else. Chakras are spinning wheels of energy located mainly along the spinal column. When they are all open and balanced, you get a free flow of energy from the base of your spine through the crown of your head. In a chakra exercise, we repeated the mantra "*Yam*" (pronounced Yah-m) at the heart chakra, and I felt tightness in my chest. For a fleeting moment I thought I was having a heart attack. Instead of panicking, though, I just allowed the experience to happen. The pressure around my heart intensified. Then I felt a pop, like the uncorking of a bottle, followed by a sputtering movement that transitioned into a steady humming sensation. That's when I realized that I had actually experienced the opening of my closed heart. I became open to the possibility that maybe I was not my physical body, which would one day die and decay. Perhaps, instead, I was the current of energy that flowed through it.

Viewing yourself as energy that can change form but never be destroyed is preferable to identifying with a decaying body as your home. We experience energy in various forms within the dream world, where everything is alterable. And anything that is alterable is not eternal.

Make no mistake: the ego can use the concept of energy for its own purpose of separation quite easily. "My formless energy is higher/purer/better than yours. I must therefore seal mine off from yours to protect and preserve the work I've done to improve myself."

The point is to be mindful about whose energy—ego's or Spirit's—is the current running through your body and heart. They are like two separate power companies. The ego's energy actually renders you powerless, and charges you dearly for it! Spirit's energy is unfailing and free. Spirit is aware that we don't actually have a separate heart in a body, but the power of love's presence *can* be experienced in our body or temporary learning device. At the point the device is no longer useful, we can experience love directly. In the meantime we can rest assured that love is infinitely better than any glimpse of it we may capture here.

LOVE IS OUR PARDON

The *Course* assures, "There is no fear in perfect love because it knows no sin, and it must look on others as on itself."[5] The flip side, or ego's script, would be "there is no love in perfect fear because it *only* knows sin, and it must look on others as on itself." Which evaluation can we trust as accurate? We either perfectly reject love in all forms without exception or we perfectly accept love in all forms without exception. The choice is between *sinful* and *sinless*.

With the ego, we're absolutely certain someone else has sinned against love and is getting what they deserve, all the while secretly believing we alone are to blame. With Spirit, we realize love cannot be destroyed, only misperceived, and a pardon for our so-called sins is automatic.

TRANQUIL AND TRIUMPHANT

Our hatred is actually long gone, but we try to keep it alive by calling upon it to darken our way. I'm always asking Spirit to show me exactly what the ego has been up to. I *really* want to uncover it all, in order to recover from it all. I've become acutely aware that we all secretly hate each other and only pretend to love, often pretending badly. The crazy part is that I'm finding this insight completely liberating and comical! It takes the guesswork out of all my relationships. I don't have to wonder if a certain person hates me . . . because they do. LOL! I don't have to wonder if I hated them first or hate them back . . . because I do. LOL!

That's what the ego is always up to, but fortunately the ego is *imaginary.* It's what I've made up to replace the truth. And at every moment that I can opt out of ego, I heal myself and others. The *Course* reveals, "The holiest of all the spots on earth is where an ancient hatred has become a present love."[6] By reminding ourselves to choose the real over the unreal, we reach a state of being that is *tranquil and triumphant.*

CHALLENGE #2

TAKE THE CHALLENGE AND BE THE CHANGE

The Source of Love is alive in our memory if we don't actively block it. This allows us to stop looking hopelessly for love within an illusory world built upon love's opposite. Remember that we could easily love everyone and everything *if we hadn't first decided to hate it.* What a bummer! It doesn't have to be that way though.

This chapter concludes with this twenty-four-hour challenge: **For today and today only, I am willing to believe that extending love is effortless.**

- I can easily extend love to the deer grazing in the yard
  because I am only love.

- I can easily extend love to the people involved in this fender bender I just passed
  because I am only love.

- I can easily extend love to this dirty floor I haven't gotten around to cleaning
  because I am only love.

- I can easily extend love to all members of
  Congress
  because I am only love.

- I can easily extend love to my middle-aged body
  because I am only love.

- I can easily extend love to the night sky full of stars
  because I am only love.

Your turn to believe that extending love is effortless.
Who or what can you extend love to today?

LIE #1

YOU CAN'T COUNT ON ANYONE BUT YOURSELF

(and, by the way,
you're a huge
disappointment)

think it's time I reveal the gift I was born with. (Don't be jealous.) *Feeling dead inside.* I used to see it as a curse, struggling with depression for most of forty years. Being raised in the Catholic faith didn't help. Getting a PhD in psychology and working with children didn't really enliven me. Chasing dreams of pop stardom while reading a small mountain of self-help books wasn't the answer either. I attribute my lasting triumph over destructive thought patterns to the study and practice of A *Course in Miracles.*

I experienced several major breakthroughs early in my *Course* study. The first was that there was nothing to *do* to overcome my problems—but much to *understand* to regain my vitality. The second was the distinction between external and internal. I'd long felt that my external self was the self I presented to the world through the roles I played, and my internal self comprised all my private thoughts of self-hatred. I came to understand that those destructive thoughts were just as external to my reality as everything else.

IF YOU DON'T HAVE ANYTHING NICE TO THINK . . .

. . . don't think anything at all! And the ego never really does. With this awareness, our mind can return to its natural state of *knowing* the truth. In other words, when we don't actively try to deny the love that we are—with the fake thoughts driven by ego—we can *feel* love's life-affirming presence move through us. The *Course* says, "Your mind holds only what you think with God. Your self-deceptions cannot take the place of truth."[1]

We don't have to search for "God thoughts," for they arise organically in the mind we share. We are only meant to stop trying to resuscitate our opposite-of-God thoughts, for they were dead on arrival in our mind, being insane and impossible in the first place. What is of God can have no opposite, and we are most certainly of God. The challenge is to see through our dream world of illusion in order to remember our divinity.

THE ISOLATION OF PERSECUTION

The ego, the fear-driven part of your mind, is out to persecute you personally. Although it's actually not personal: it reserves the same fate for all of us to take the idea of separation to the extreme where we each experience the horror of not feeling connected to a single thing. And the ego won't rest until it gets you to that place of suffering in solitary confinement.

The key to the kingdom of God (love) is to remember that we never left it. It's actually arrogant to believe we could! The *Course* implores us to see the kingdom we invented for what it really is: our personal version of hell. "You think you are the home of evil, darkness and sin."[2] Because we accept this ego-given "truth" on an unconscious level, we think, feel, and act in accordance with that lie.

At a retreat I attended recently, we did a group meditation with the intent of looking at the ego head-on, a shared willingness to see all of it. What came to me out of the silence was a variation of a Catholic prayer, *The Gloria*, that I remember reciting as a child. The actual lines from the prayer, referring to Jesus, were: *You alone are the Holy One. You alone are the Most High*. And I immediately felt that I was, by comparison, the polar opposite: *I alone am the sinner. I alone am the most low*. I experienced an impassable chasm between these states in my mind, and there was no one else to blame. It was all squarely on me, and the thought of it was crushing.

LET'S FINALIZE
(releasing the need to further analyze)

Post-traumatic stress disorder (PTSD) occurs following the experience of a life-threatening event that invokes feelings of helplessness or intense fear. In our existential predicament, the key is to acknowledge that we *are* afraid for our lives. We're terrified of retaliation from our Source over the destruction of perfect oneness as a result of our decision to separate from it. It's equivalent to pressing the "nuke button." The ego, the idea that the separation/mass murder actually happened, was born out of this trauma. Too painful to face up close, the ego was projected outward in the making or imagining of the world to serve as an elaborate hiding spot where others could be blamed for evils I secretly felt I alone had done. And fear of being found out is inescapable.

When we give power to the images we've made—by investing our belief—we follow the ego's descent into madness. It was Robert Jay Lifton's work on the psychological impact of war that eventually led to the addition of PTSD as a recognized anxiety disorder. In his book *Home from the War*, he wrote, "In such an inverted moral universe, whatever residual ethical sensitivity impels the individual against adjusting to evil is under constant external *and internal* assault." But aren't we all in this very situation? We are forced under pressure to "adjust to evil" when we align with the ego.

Spirit gently reminds us that we are under no coercion but our own and speaks to us in a language we can understand to undo our murder mentality. Spirit confirms that we *do* believe we've murdered each other. And we essentially have when we see others as separate from us. To see others as separate is to see them as they are not now, never have been, and never will be. It *is* a "murder" or complete negation of who they really are—indestructible and eternal as One. Spirit encourages us to take this a step further and realize that the same holds true for our Source. We did not, in fact, accomplish the impossible. Perfect oneness could never be destroyed. It turns out that the only thing that was separate was our "nuke button," in the sense that it was not connected to anything and had no real effects at all!

THE LUXURY BOX OF PAIN

We can't move beyond the pain as long as we harbor an actual unconscious *desire* to keep it, based on the assumption that it's well deserved. In his book *Ending Our Escape from Love*, Ken Wapnick says, "We would all agree that pain is something we do not want, but if we were to look at what is going on in our minds, we would realize that we in fact luxuriate in the pain."

It's like we reserved the luxury box at a sporting event, although it's a luxury box full of torture devices! This is something we can't afford to keep, not if we are serious about wanting love, peace, and joy in its place. Unshakeable peace is a goal more realistic than we ever thought possible. We have to root for it though, like it's our home team. The visiting team is the ego, and we can decide that it has worn out its welcome. Although it came by our invitation, it has destroyed everything in its path and it plays for keeps. It's an unwinnable game, and it's time to call it quits.

I've heard myself say out loud that I have a high tolerance for pain, as if it was a badge of honor or a sign of strength. I see now that it's a sign of ego strength. I was referring to physical pain, but all physical pain can be traced back to mental pain. The treatment prescribed by Spirit is twofold:

1. Understand that you're never in pain for the reason you think. Our pain seems to be inflicted upon us by something external, but it's always self-inflicted. It's the internal, unconscious trauma of believing we permanently cut ourselves off from our Source of Love, like a fresh-cut rose in a vase. It appears to have life apart from its source of nourishment for a time, but it's on borrowed time and will inevitably wither and die.

2. Decide that you are willing to experience how things really are with the Teacher of love by your side. This decision *can't fail* unless you change your mind and default back to the teacher of pain.

You'll know you're following the right teacher with at least some consistency when periods of pure anguish become few and far between. When I was in the midst of postpartum depression, I not only cried several times during the day, I also would often wake up with matted eyelashes and a wet pillow from crying in my sleep. There was not even a slight interruption in my suffering. Now it's the other way around. I only experience slight interruptions in my peace. I attribute this shift to a change in perception from fear to love, though I'm certainly not done!

BECOMING A CONSISTENT LOVE CHOOSER

Thought by thought, we can learn to choose wisely—sorting the false from the true and the fearful from the loving—and enjoy the positive results. We have to maintain awareness that we even have a choice, which is not always easy. The ego always speaks first and loudest, while Spirit is the quiet alternative. Spirit will always be the choice that brings clarity and unity. With the ego, we settle for chaos and divisiveness.

The *Course* instructs, "How can you know whether you chose the stairs to heaven or the way to hell? Quite easily. How do you feel?"[3] Any time we feel less than magnificent, we know we've chosen hell. Choice precedes feeling without exception. Therefore, focusing your attention on the level of thought where *you* make decisions is crucial to success.

If you feel okay, it doesn't necessarily follow that you've chosen correctly, for the ego has grown very skilled at making us feel somewhat good. But the good feeling of transcending fear is very different than the sort-of-good feeling that derives from burying fear so deep that it can't even surface for examination. How can you tell the difference? If the peace you feel involves extending love to everyone without exception, you can trust it. But if the peace is conditional in any way, dependent on things working out for you but not so much for others, then you can bet it's an ego trap.

LAUGH YOUR WAY OUT OF IT

It would serve us well to remember to laugh as much as possible. When we find ourselves caught in an ego trap, laughing is the quickest way out of it. The ego is always encouraging us to gravitate toward negative emotions that block our natural state of permanent joy. But you may be wondering, isn't it healthy to express any emotion that comes up? After all, we're only human. To that I would say, "Not really. And are you sure?"

I remember an experience I had with my son Gavin a few years back. I was yelling at him for something he had done or failed to do; I can't remember which. He just looked at me calmly and said, "So much for inner peace, Mom." And then we laughed together. Accepting a negative emotion as a possible state of being (as in "I'm angry!") is only healthy to the ego. It uses negative emotions like vitamin supplements meant to prolong its life.

The ego's days are numbered though. It is the only part of us that can die, and this is because it was never really a part of us. To remember this truth, we only need give the teacher of misery the pink slip, and its curriculum of death—rooted in the world of illusion—will go along with it. The new hire, the Teacher of joy, asks, "Can we laugh about it yet?" The *Course* suggests, "The world will end in laughter, because it is a place of tears. Where there is laughter, who can longer weep?"[4]

IT'S AN EXERCISE
(mental stretching required)

We won't let ourselves out of the imprisonment of isolation as long as we think we're unworthy of release. To be more specific, the ego wants us to judge ourselves and reach the conclusion that we are nothing good and everything faulty. In an attempt to survive this crushing judgment, we figure out that the only way to escape it is to project faults on to others. We try to convince ourselves that shortcomings are not applicable to us, when all the while we secretly believe they absolutely are true.

Spirit tells us that what we project on to others we have not escaped. We've just held it away from ourselves and kept it hidden where it can't be healed. It's really a continuum, where perceiving that all faults are only in others is reflective of an intense fear that the opposite is true. Seeing some faults in others and claiming a few reveals a willingness to identify the source of them. Claiming all faults as my own, in the sense that I made them up to secure my belief in my fundamental unworthiness, is associated with a tremendous willingness to heal. And the healed state is not to believe that faults serve any purpose or are even possible.

Most of us are in the "keep a few/dish out a few" stage. Which faults of the ego would you say are true of you sometimes, and which would trigger a defensive reaction from you in the form of "That's not me at all!"? I'll go first.

Ego Faults from A to Z	Sometimes true of me	NEVER true of me
Aggressive, Boring, Cynical, Dishonest, Eccentric, Foolish, Gullible, Harsh, Impulsive, Jealous, Kitschy, Lazy, Moody, Narrow-minded, Obsessive, Pessimistic, Quick-tempered, Resentful, Stupid, Thoughtless, Unreliable, Vain, Weak-willed, Xenophobic, Yielding, (Over)Zealous	1. cynical 2. moody 3. obsessive 4. yielding	1. boring 2. lazy 3. narrow-minded 4. stupid

If anyone were to refer to me as anything from my "Sometimes true of me" list, I'd reluctantly agree and would probably be mildly insulted, but I truly feel that I could *Shake it Off* like the Taylor Swift song. From my "Never true of me" list, being called *stupid* would definitely trigger the strongest reaction from me in the form of defensiveness. Now, it's your turn to identify your triggers from the list of empty ego insults, and then we'll undo them together. This is not an exhaustive list, just a starting point. Feel free to add to it if you'd like. You can also list more than four insults in each category. Maybe nearly everything on the list triggers you. Just be honest with your reactions. Honesty brings about transformation.

Ego Insults from A to Z	Sometimes true of me	NEVER true of me
Aggressive, Boring, Cynical, Dishonest, Eccentric, Foolish, Gullible, Harsh, Impulsive, Jealous, Kitschy, Lazy, Moody, Narrow-minded, Obsessive, Pessimistic, Quick-tempered, Resentful, Stupid, Thoughtless, Unreliable, Vain, Weak-willed, Xenophobic, Yielding, (Over)Zealous	1. _____ 2. _____ 3. _____ 4. _____	1. _____ 2. _____ 3. _____ 4. _____

I can see now, after decades of reflection, that when I defend *against* something, I give it tremendous power over me. Could it be that the very reason for my worldly existence is to prove I'm not stupid? I remember the first time I got all A's on my report card in fifth grade. I told myself that if I could do it once, I must do it always. Whichever label was the most cringe-worthy for you serves the same purpose: keeping you stuck in the belief that your worth is up for grabs and must be defended. Possibly, while caught up in defensiveness, we turned away from the solution that required the opposite. Spirit says that defenselessness is our true nature, for nothing real requires defending. Our perfection *is* real. But we defend against it out of disbelief, saying, "It just can't be true!" We experience this perfection when we shift away from seeking outer proof of its existence in the world and look inward where it can be known as a constant state.

DON'T FORGET TO CLAIM YOUR TREASURE

I recently had a dream of exploring a cave and finding a treasure chest full of jewels. To me this symbolized that we are rewarded greatly for making the journey way down within. Specifically, we are rewarded with abundance that was previously concealed. It's not a worldly treasure but rather a direct connection to what lies beyond the world.

Each individual jewel is like a recovered memory of our true and eternal identity as One.

The *Course* instructs: "Give thanks to every part of you that you have taught to remember you."[5] Gratitude grows in intensity incrementally as we willfully and joyfully surrender our false identity for the one we could never lose. Trusting that no fallout will result hastens our progress.

It's like the experience we all had as children waiting for the prize at the bottom of the cereal box. We don't have to ingest every nutrient-poor piece of cereal (our ego thoughts) between us and the prize. We can just tip over the box and get right to it instead! It's not cheating; it's an effective spiritual strategy. We can save time, not to mention the existential stomach ache caused by chewing through all our delusions. That process can take a very long time, but it doesn't have to take any time at all. The "prize" is ours for the taking right now. It is the magnificence of our true identity in Spirit, and it comes with the knowledge that we may appear to be in the dream world, the ego's playground, but we are not of it.

LIVING THE HAPPY DREAM

The goal we share is to awaken from the dream of fear completely. It's too big a leap, though, to awaken directly from a nightmare. You've probably experienced an intense startling response waking up from a nightmare, when you have to wait for your heart to stop pounding before you can fall back asleep. Spirit helps make this transition easier for us. Joy is allowed! We will experience a temporary dream of joy until we can seamlessly connect to the real, eternal bliss beyond the dream.

You'll know you're making progress in remembering what you really are—love and nothing else—when typical triggers lose their power. It's not an attitude of "I don't care." It's rather that your caring extends equally to everyone and it's therefore much harder to get upset at anyone in particular. The dark cloud of fear is lifting, and you can't help but see the light cast on everyone.

It's helpful not to attach to the form of the dream by saying, "It has to look this way for me." There may be forms of joy we'd prefer to have, but with the Teacher of love as our guide, we can work with anything. When I was living in Los Angeles, pursuing my dream of becoming a pop star, I shadowed celebrities like it was a part-time job. I thought I would feel elevated as a result of it. Now I know that feeling is a state of mind. That is, I can feel just as high dancing by myself at home in my pajamas as I did that time I danced on stage with Snoop Dogg at the club White Lotus in Hollywood.

The point is to dance for the joy of it, like no one is watching or judging—which is true. For there is only One of us here appearing as many! All judgment is self-judgment. Viewing the body as an imaginary border between us helps us in the reassembly that must take place in the mind. The pursuit of only wanting to experience our oneness will help us transcend any fleeting experience of isolation. We could never be alone, even if we wanted to be. And we don't want to be!

TAKE THE CHALLENGE AND BE THE CHANGE

It all comes down to understanding that either everything the ego says is true or everything Spirit says is true. At no point do their views intersect. A choice, or pledge of allegiance, must be made. The stakes may seem high, and they certainly would be if there actually was a choice to make. But only one option is real, which means we can't get it wrong!

We've covered the top ten lies of the ego, but there are legions more. Spirit only speaks for truth, for it is truth, as are we. With Spirit guidance, we can exchange everything we thought we were for everything we actually are. We are not defective but perfect. We are not alone but One. We are not perishable but eternal. The acceptance of this revelation results in the experience of all-encompassing peace. It is constant, and no one is excluded. It cannot fail, for it is directly connected to our Source of peace.

The twenty-four-hour challenge for this chapter: **For today and today only, I am willing to believe that peace is constant.**

- My husband forgot to stop at Costco on his way home, but my peace is constant.
- The kids rushed through their homework again, but my peace is constant.

- Someone misunderstood my Facebook post completely, but my peace is constant.
- It may be time to start using my inhaler again, but my peace is constant.
- Not one positive event was mentioned on the evening news, but my peace is constant.
- The skies are overcast, but my peace is constant.

. . . And all is well.

How can you practice your belief that peace is constant?

ACKNOWLEDGMENTS

First, I'd like to acknowledge my own perseverance in seeing this project through to the end of the five years it took to complete it. I have to give credit to the guidance I've learned to trust. To my husband, my biggest supporter, I sincerely thank you for allowing me to publicly unravel my fears, and remembering that only my most loving thoughts are true. I'm grateful to my children for giving me a daily dose of lighthearted joy. Thank you, Dad, Mom, Andy, and Lisa—the cast of characters in my childhood home. I wouldn't change a single thing. I'm also blessed to have such amazing friends in my life, including my companions at Greenlight Sanctuaries ACIM Group (on Facebook): John & Lainie Beavin, Myrna Smith, and Jack O'Neill.

To my agent and editor, D. Patrick Miller, I credit you with helping me find my voice and infusing me with confidence, and for introducing me to my spirit sisters at Fearless Books & Literary Services: Maria Felipe, Corinne Zupko, and Lyna Rose. Thanks to Jon Mundy, for being the first to publish my work in *Miracles Magazine*; David Fishman, for helping me build a platform on ACIM *Gather Radio*; and Gary Renard, for demonstrating a laughter-infused teaching style that I've tried to adopt. And endless gratitude to Nora Rawn, my editor at Ixia Press, for believing in this book and for her valuable insight along the way, as well as to the entire team at Dover Publications. Cover photo credit to my friends Chris Polacco of Picture Perfect Designer Photography and Stephanie Alami, makeup artist extraordinaire.

I'd also like to deeply thank anyone who takes the time to join with me in reading this book. Together, we can demonstrate that we simply have no use for fear.

Choose love and be love. . . .

INDEX OF REFERENCES

All quotes from A *Course in Miracles* are from the third edition, published in 2007. They are used with written permission from the copyright holder and publisher, the Foundation for Inner Peace, PO Box 598, Mill Valley, California 94942-0598, www.acim.org and info@acim.org.

For this index, please follow the examples below to correspond with the numbering system used in A *Course in Miracles*.

T-26.IV.4:7 = Text, Chapter 26, Section IV, Paragraph 4, Sentence 7.

W-pl.169.5:2 = Workbook, Part 1, Lesson 169, Paragraph 5, Sentence 2.

M-13.3:2 = Manual, Question 13, Paragraph 3, Sentence 2.

C-6.4:6 = Clarification of Terms, Term 6, Paragraph 4, Sentence 6.

P-2.VI.5:1 = Psychotherapy, Chapter 2, Section 6, Paragraph 5, Sentence 1.

S-1.V.4:3 = Song of Prayer, Chapter 1, Section 5, Paragraph 4, Sentence 3.

INTRODUCTION

1. T-27.VIII.6:2

LIE #10

1. T-29.VII.1:9   2. T-21.II.5:1   3. T-21.VIII.1:1   4. T-21.VIII.1:3-4

LIE #9

1. T-19.IV-D.12:8   2. T-21.In.1:4   3. T-22.In.4:8
4. W-P2.13.5:1

LIE #8

1. W-P1.Rev-V-In.4:2   2. M-17.7:11   3. W-P1.189.7:1-3
4. W-P1.191.2:4   5. T-4.VI.3:3   6. T-24.III.3:1-2

LIE #7

1. T-12.IV.1:4   2. T-16.IV.2:1   3. T-16.IV.1:1   4. T-17.IV.2:6
5. T-18.VI.9:10   6. T-16.IV.11:3-4

LIE #6

1. W-PI.152.11:1   2. T-24.I.4:4   3. T-24.I.6:5   4. T-24.I.9:1-2
5. T-16.VI.8:1-2

LIE #5

1. T-13.XI.2:2-3   2. T-13.I.1:4   3. T-31.VIII.6:2   4. M-16.6:9-11
5. W-PI.107.5:2

LIE #4

1. W-PI.85.1:2   2. W-PI.140.3:2-3   3. T-23.IV.9:5
4. T-30.VI.2:8   5. M-3.1:1   6. W-P2.249.1:1

LIE #3

1. T-5.In.2:2   2. T-30.VII.3:8-9   3. T-11.VIII.13:3   4. T-7.VI.4:5

LIE #2

1. W-PI.117.2:2   2. T-12.V.6:1-3   3. T-24.I.1:3-4
4. W-PI.127.1:3-5   5. T-20.III.11:3   6. T-26.IX.6:1

LIE #1

1. W-PI.Rev-IV-In.4:1-2   2. W-PI.93.1:1   3. T-23.II.22:6-8
4. M-14.5:5-6   5. T-13.VII.17:8

ABOUT THE AUTHOR

Dana Marrocco is a writer, motivational speaker, singer/songwriter, and self-help stand-up comedian. She lives with her family in New Jersey. She received a PhD in educational psychology from Purdue University, specializing in theories of learning and motivation. Dr. Dana has recently published articles in *Elephant Journal* and *Miracles Magazine*. Before focusing exclusively on self-help, she was published in major professional journals in her field of educational psychology.

As a motivational speaker, Dr. Dana presents regularly at churches and retreats across the country, often in the form of musical skits mixed with lectures. Her dynamic comedic delivery is consistently well received with attendee comments such as "You are just what this conference needed. I was about to fall asleep before you came on!" Her unique style of delivery is reflected in the YouTube series "Did You Forget to Laugh?" She recently won an award for a song parody performance from *Noisey*. In addition, she holds a weekly teaching spot on ACIM *Gather Radio* and performs original music with her band, Dr. Dana and the Infinite Patients.

Connect with Dr. Dana at www.drdanamarrocco.com and @drdanamarrocco.